The
Clinical
Placement

An essential guide for nursing students 3e

**Tracy
Levett-Jones**

Sharon Bourgeois

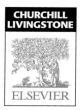

CHURCHILL
LIVINGSTONE

ELSEVIER

Sydney   Edinburgh   London   New York   Philadelphia   St Louis   Toronto

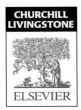

is an imprint of Elsevier

Elsevier Australia. ACN 001 002 357
(a division of Reed International Books Australia Pty Ltd)
Tower 1, 475 Victoria Avenue, Chatswood, NSW 2067

This edition © 2015 Elsevier Australia. Reprinted 2015

National Library of Australia Cataloguing-in-Publication Data

---

9780729542012

Levett-Jones, Tracy, author.

The clinical placement / Tracy Levett-Jones, Sharon Bourgeois.
3rd edition.
9780729542012 (paperback)
Nursing—Textbooks.
Nursing—Study and teaching (Higher)
Bourgeois, Sharon, author.

610.73

Content Strategist: Libby Houston
Content Development Specialists: Vicky Spichopoulos and Tamsin Curtis
Project manager: Anitha Rajarathnam
Edited by Matt Davies
Proofread by Kate Stone
Cover and internal design by Lisa Petroff
Index by Robert Swanson
Typeset by Toppan Best-set Premedia Limited
Printed in China by 1010 Printing International Limited

Cover and text images from: iStockphoto.com, 07-25-11 © sturti, iStockphoto.com, 12-05-11 © DOUGBERRY, iStockphoto.com, 07-12-10 © DarrenMower, iStockphoto.com, 10-13-11 © annedde, iStockphoto.com, 05-03-11 © francisblack, iStockphoto.com, 12-13-10 © milandarula, iStockphoto.com, 04-17-12 © francisblack, iStockphoto.com, 03-28-11 © AlexRaths

CONTENTS

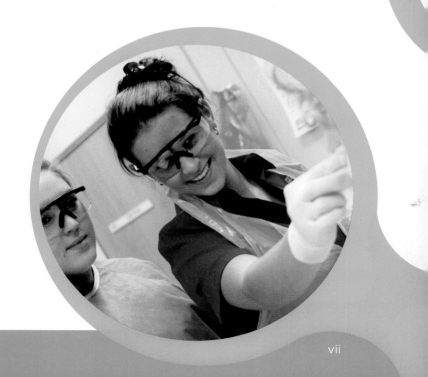

DEDICATIONS

To the amazing nursing students whose journeys into nursing I have had the privilege of sharing; and to Tyler Alexander Jones, with love.

Tracy Levett-Jones

I dedicate this book to all students of nursing (past, present and future): a genuine treasure to human kind.
To Patrice, my heartfelt thanks for your support; you are always there.

Sharon Bourgeois

A special thanks to the University of Wollongong for providing images used on the cover and in the table of contents.

ABOUT THE AUTHORS

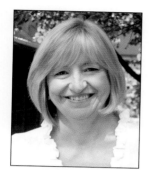

Professor Tracy Levett-Jones
PhD, MEd & Work BN, DipAppSC(Nsg), RN

Tracy is the Deputy Head of School (Teaching and Learning) in the School of Nursing and Midwifery and the Director of the Research Centre for Health Professional Education at the University of Newcastle. Her research interests include clinical education, belongingness, clinical reasoning, simulation, interprofessional education, cultural competence and patient safety. Tracy's doctoral research explored the clinical learning experiences of students in Australia and the United Kingdom. She has a broad clinical background and, prior to her academic career, worked as a medical-surgical nurse and nurse educator. Tracy has authored a number of books, book chapters and journal papers on clinical education and has received 10 teaching and learning awards, which include a New South Wales Minister for Education Quality Teaching Award and an Australian Learning and Teaching Council Award for Teaching Excellence.

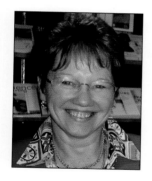

Associate Professor Sharon Bourgeois
PhD, MEd, MA, BA, OT Cert, FCNA, RN

Sharon works with staff and students on the School of Nursing outreach campuses (Bega, Batemans Bay, Shoalhaven, Southern Sydney) at the University of Wollongong. There, she lectures in both the undergraduate and the postgraduate programs of nursing and is recognised as a teaching scholar for the school. Sharon has been involved in various leadership roles associated with nursing education, facilitating students' clinical and theoretical learning and supporting registered nurses' educational development. Her formal research interests have focused on the discourses of caring—identifying 'an archive of caring for nursing'. She has a strong interest in models of education and students' experiences of the clinical learning environment. Sharon's nursing experiences began in New Zealand as a student nurse. This was followed by clinical experiences in surgical, general practice, perioperative nursing and education in both New Zealand and Australia. In 2009 Sharon was the recipient of the Vice Chancellor's Award for Teaching Excellence at the University of Western Sydney. She advocates that nurses embrace all elements of the professional role to enhance and promote care.

REVIEWERS

Maree Bauld MEd, MCN, Grad Cert L&T HlthProf, GradDip CritCare, RN
Lecturer, School of Health Sciences, University of Tasmania, Launceston, Tasmania,
Australia

Jan Edwards BAppSc, GradDip(Ed), MPHC, PhD, FACN, CENA, AWMA, RM, RN
Lecturer, School of Health Professions, Murdoch University, Perth, Western Australia,
Australia

Liz James BLibS, MEd, RM, RN
Midwifery Team Manager, Centre for Health and Social Practice, Waikato Institute of
Technology, Hamilton, New Zealand
New Zealand College of Midwives

Carley Jans BA(Nsg), MAEd
Lecturer, University of Wollongong at SMART Infrastructure Facility, Wollongong,
New South Wales, Australia

Victoria Kain NICC, PhD, MN, RN
Senior Lecturer, School of Nursing and Midwifery, Griffith University, Gold Coast,
Queensland, Australia

Kylie Russell PhD, MA HScEd, BA(Nsg)
Clinical Coordinator, School of Nursing and Midwifery, The University of Notre Dame,
Fremantle, Western Australia, Australia

Christine Taylor PhD, MHScEd, BSc(Hons), BAppSc(AdvNsg), RN
Senior Lecturer, School of Nursing and Midwifery, University of Western Sydney,
Penrith, New South Wales, Australia
Executive Committee Member, Australian Nurse Teachers' Society

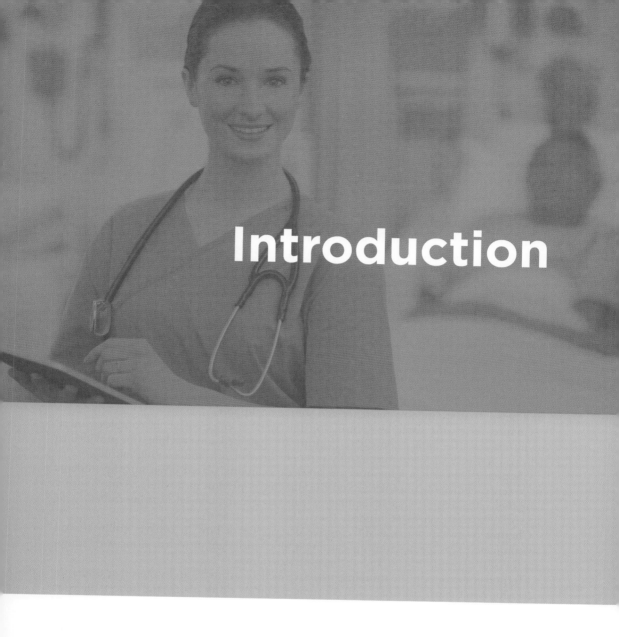

Introduction

The aim of this book is to guide you on your clinical journey. There is plenty of evidence—anecdotal and empirical—to suggest that clinical placement experiences can be both tremendous and challenging. This book will help you to appreciate and capitalise on the tremendous, and to ride out any challenging situations you may encounter, in what is sure to be one of the most exciting journeys of your life.

The ultimate goal of clinical education is to develop nurses who are confident and competent beginning practitioners. Positive and productive clinical placement experiences are pivotal to your success. This book encourages you to use your clinical placements as opportunities to develop the skills, knowledge and understandings that underpin quality practice, and to appreciate the clinical environment for the wonderful learning experience that it is.

This book explores both the complex issues and the everyday situations that make up clinical placements. Although it is written primarily for nursing students, it will also be of interest to anyone involved in the clinical education of undergraduate nurses or new graduates. Academics, clinical educators, facilitators, clinicians, mentors and managers will find the information it contains useful as a stimulus for dialogue and debate in tutorials, inservices and debriefing sessions. The book's interactive style is designed to engage with active readers and to encourage them to integrate the material into their practice. Some of the sections are deliberately provocative in order to challenge your assumptions and preconceptions and to help you think more critically about important issues.

HOW TO USE THIS BOOK

Each chapter consists of a number of different sections. Within these sections theory is interwoven to explain core principles. **Learning activities** appear throughout the book to help you relate theory to the reality of practice. **'Something to think about' boxes** provide words of wisdom to reflect on, and valuable snippets of advice. **Coaching tips** allow you to apply what you learn to your clinical experiences. **Student stories** and reflections bring the book to life and will encourage you to re-examine your own practice experiences.

Students who have read earlier editions of this book provide the following advice: Read Chapters 1–3 early in your nursing program, before you attend any clinical placements. These chapters provide foundational knowledge that will set you up to be successful. Read Chapters 4 and 5 thoughtfully—they are written at a more sophisticated level and are deliberately designed to challenge you to excel as a nurse. Most students read these chapters before they attend a placement but continue to use them throughout their nursing program (and beyond) as an ongoing reference and source of support.

Chapter 1 sets the scene by focusing on the 'rules of engagement' in complex clinical environments. The clinical context and culture are described and coaching tips provided to help you navigate your way successfully through this dynamic and exciting journey.

Chapter 2 provides insights into the 'great expectations' placed upon nursing students by patients, clinicians, universities and the nursing profession as a whole. Armed with a clear understanding of what is required as you traverse the clinical learning milieu, your chances of success will be multiplied.

Chapter 3 gives a practical and positive description of how to behave within clinical environments. Tips for maximising learning opportunities are provided, along with strategies for dealing with difficult and challenging situations.

Chapter 4 focuses on the thinking processes, beliefs, attitudes and values that underpin successful clinical performance and encourages you to think about and reflect on your experiences in ways that are meaningful and relevant.

Chapter 5 looks at the ways nurses define and promote their profession through effective communication and gives advice on how to interact with patients and colleagues in ways that are both person-centred and clinically safe.

In this book our role as 'storytellers' has been made possible by borrowing experiences from many people. We would like to thank the many generous students and colleagues who have shared their stories and insights with us.

Since the first edition of our book was published in 2007 we have received a great deal of positive feedback from reviewers and students alike. Comments such as those below have affirmed the value of our book as a guide to clinical placement:

'I felt like your book was written just for me, I couldn't put it down—I read it from cover to cover in one sitting.'

'I just used your book again in another assignment. I'm sure putting a book like this together is a labour of love and I just wanted you to know that it's like having a mate on hand for the times when you are really questioning your placement experiences.'

'This book is GREAT!! It validates everything we have been trying to get across to students. It is becoming a prescribed text from this minute!'

'I love your book. I showed it to the students and encouraged them all to get one, told them it was full of great info and interesting stories ... it's a masterpiece!'

'I have added this book to our library; it is invaluable for our educators.'

In this version we have retained much of the original, but we have enhanced the sections that address contemporary issues such as patient safety, clinical reasoning, therapeutic communication, interprofessional communication and the use of social media (to name a few). We hope you enjoy (and learn from) our latest edition and that it helps you achieve success in your nursing journey.

CLINICAL PLACEMENT INSIGHTS

The 'Insights from experts' chapter from previous editions of this book is now an exciting compilation of videos where clinicians introduce you to the learning opportunities provided in diverse practice areas. Although we haven't been able to cover every clinical specialty, the selection we have included will open your eyes to the wonderful opportunities available to nursing students and to graduates.

To access the videos go to <http://evolve.elsevier.com/AU/Levett-Jones/placement/>. Note: The stories included in this book are real, but the names have been changed to maintain confidentiality.

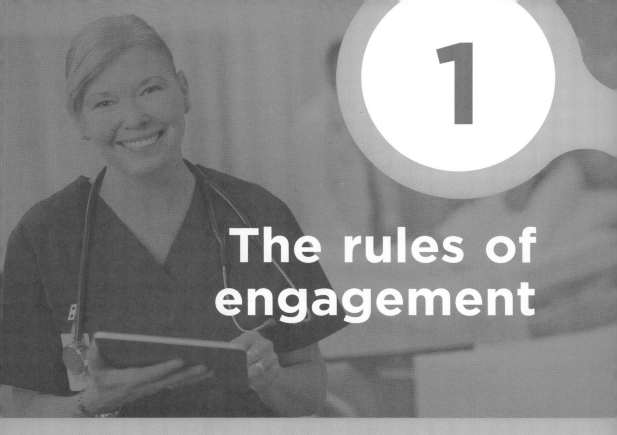

1

The rules of engagement

Every one of us receives and passes on an inheritance. The inheritance may not be an accumulation of earthly possessions or acquired riches, but whether we realize it or not, our choices, words, actions, and values will impact someone and form the heritage we hand down.

Ben Hardesty—musician

INTRODUCTION
In this chapter we introduce you to the social and professional world of nursing and the key people you will encounter on clinical placements. We share some of the hidden assumptions and understandings that underlie clinical practice and clinical cultures. In essence, this chapter provides insight into what makes contemporary practice so dynamic, challenging and exciting. It will help you find your 'place' in clinical practice environments and equip you to work effectively with nurses and other health professionals.

KNOW THE LIE OF THE LAND
Over the past two decades healthcare environments have become increasingly complex, technological, consumer-oriented and litigious. Factors such as high patient throughput,

increased acuity and decreased length of stay mean that people who are hospitalised are sicker than ever before and stay in hospital for increasingly shorter periods of time. When coupled with nursing shortages and variations in skill mix, these factors have made the working lives of nurses in acute care environments increasingly demanding, exciting and sometimes stressful. Additionally, with the increased focus on health promotion and illness prevention, more and more nurses are choosing to work in community and primary health-care settings, and their roles have expanded in scope and responsibility (Department of Health and Ageing 2010).

We share this information at the beginning of the book to prepare you for the journey ahead. It would be risky to travel to a foreign land without some degree of preparation in order to develop an understanding of the people, culture and context. The clinical learning environment is no different. Without an understanding of all that nursing in the contemporary healthcare contexts means, you may find yourself confused by the dichotomy between what you think nurses and nursing should be and what they actually are.

As the challenges and expectations associated with clinical nursing have increased, so too have the rewards, the satisfaction and the sheer joy of knowing you have made a real difference to people's lives. You will be inspired as you observe committed nurses providing safe and effective patient care despite the clinical challenges they encounter. This book will help you prepare for your journey into this dynamic and exciting clinical environment.

Coaching tips

- The first step in preparing for your journey into the clinical placement is to make sure you are familiar with your university's expectations, guidelines, procedures, policies and contact people.
- The second step (of course) is to read this book!

THE CLINICAL PLACEMENT—WHAT IT IS AND WHY IT MATTERS

Clinical placements (sometimes called clinical practicum, work-integrated learning, professional placements or workplace experiences) are where the world of nursing comes alive. You will learn how nurses think, feel and behave, what they value and how they communicate. You will come to understand the culture and ethos of nursing in contemporary practice, as well as the complexities and challenges nurses encounter. Some students say that clinical placements change the way they view the world. Whether this is true for you will depend, to a large extent, on how you approach it. Most importantly, clinical placements provide opportunities to engage with and care for clients, to enter their world and to establish meaningful therapeutic relationships.

Clinical learning

Competent nurses have a significant impact upon the people and communities they serve. Quality nursing care results in reductions in patient mortality and critical incidents, such

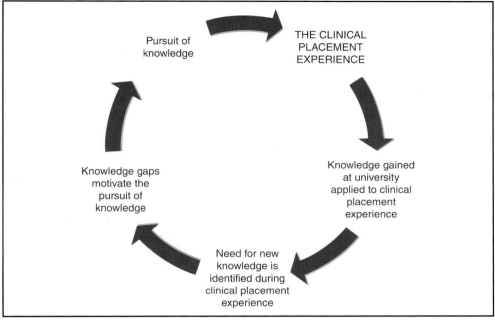

Figure 1.1 The cyclical nature of knowledge pursuit and clinical application

as medication errors, patient falls, hospital-acquired infections and pressure ulcers (Desai et al. 2013; Karavasiliadou & Athanasakis 2014; Reid-Searl et al. 2010; Tran & Johnson 2010). Clinical placements are where you apply the knowledge gained through your academic pursuits to the reality of practice and by doing so learn to make a positive difference to the health and wellbeing of the people you care for. Additionally, analysis and critical reflection on your clinical learning experiences will make the areas in which you need more knowledge and experience apparent. In this way knowledge pursuit and clinical application become an ongoing cycle of learning (see Figure 1.1).

Clinical placement patterns

Depending on where you study, your clinical placement patterns will vary. Your placements may be scheduled in a 'block' pattern, in which you attend for a week or longer at a time; you may attend on regular days each week or you may have a combination of attendance patterns.

Clinical placement settings

Clinical placements occur across a broad range of practice settings and vary depending on where you study and according to the approved program of study. Each clinical area has inherent learning opportunities. Typically, you can expect to undertake placements in some or all of these areas:

- community and primary healthcare settings
- medical/surgical units (e.g. cardiac, respiratory, urology, orthopaedics, haematology)

- critical care units (e.g. emergency departments, coronary care units, operating theatres, renal dialysis, intensive care units, high dependency units)
- older person services
- mental health services
- maternal and child health services
- disability services
- Aboriginal medical services
- rural and remote health settings
- public and private health facilities.

In the 'Insights from Experts' videos, nursing experts from a range of clinical practice areas share their insights about clinical practice. They each provide an overview of their context of practice, the unique learning opportunities available and the preparation required.

The videos can be viewed via the Evolve website at <http://evolve.elsevier.com/AU/Levett-Jones/placement/>.

As a complement to clinical placements, and to promote patient safety, most universities also provide simulation experiences. Through these valuable and authentic learning opportunities you will:

- be actively involved in challenging clinical situations that involve unpredictable, simulated patient deterioration
- be exposed to time-sensitive and critical clinical scenarios that, if encountered in a 'real' clinical environment, you could normally only observe
- have opportunities to apply and synthesise knowledge in a realistic but non-threatening environment
- make mistakes and learn from them without risk to patients, yourself or others
- develop your technical and non-technical skills in a safe environment
- be provided with formative and summative feedback
- enhance your learning through reflection and remediation.

PERSON-CENTRED CARE

At this early stage in the book it is important to acknowledge that nursing, and therefore clinical placements, are focused primarily on the *people for whom we care*. Everything else should take second place. For this reason we now turn to a discussion of person (or patient) -centred care.

Recognition that person-centred care is the most important attribute of patient safety has changed the landscape of contemporary healthcare (Levett-Jones et al. 2014). 'Person-centred care' is a term that has become prevalent in healthcare over the past two decades. It is a concept that nurses value highly, particularly in increasingly complex and busy clinical environments. There are various definitions of the term 'person-centred care', with each underpinned by principles such as trust, empathy, dignity, autonomy, respect, choice, transparency and the desire to help individuals lead the life they want. Person-centred care is built on the understanding that people bring their own experiences, skills and knowledge about their condition and illness. It is a holistic approach to the planning, delivery and evaluation of healthcare that is grounded in mutually beneficial partnerships between healthcare professionals, patients and families. Person-centred care applies to people of all ages and can be practised in any healthcare setting (Institute for Patient- and Family-Centered Care 2008).

Person-centred care is integrated through and underpinned by the Nursing and Midwifery Board of Australia (NMBA) and New Zealand Nursing Council professional standards and codes of practice. For example, nurses:

- respect the dignity, culture, ethnicity, values and beliefs of people receiving care and treatment, and of their colleagues (NMBA 2008)
- determine agreed priorities for resolving health needs of individuals/groups (NMBA 2006).

When health professionals, patients and families work in partnership, the quality and safety of healthcare rise, costs decrease and provider and patient satisfaction are enhanced (Levett-Jones et al. 2014). When person-centred care is integrated throughout the system there is a decrease in medical errors, readmission rates, infection rates and mortality rates, as well as a shorter average length of stay (Meterko et al. 2010; Institute for Patient- and Family-Centered Care 2008). In the care of patients with chronic conditions, studies also indicate that person-centred care reduces anxiety and improves quality of life (Bauman et al. 2003; Levinson et al. 2010).

Person-centred care involves seeing the person—not just the patient, client or resident (see Box 1.1 for an explanation of these terms). Just as being a nursing student is only one aspect of who you are, being a patient, resident or client is only one dimension of person-hood. Nurses who practise in a person-centred way recognise patients' freedom to make their own decisions as a fundamental and inalienable human right; this includes people who are experiencing mental illness or cognitive changes such as dementia.

The language used to describe the people for whom we care is often indicative of the extent to which our practice is person-centred. For example, by referring to a person as 'the bowel resection in room 23' or 'the one with dementia', their personhood becomes under-valued and they become no more than their disease, their symptoms or a task that has to be attended to.

While person-centred care may sometimes seem to be an unrealistic goal amid the busy-ness that characterises much of contemporary healthcare, it is not just another task. It is a way of being with another, of upholding their dignity, and interacting in a meaningful and memorable way.

Person-centred care also refers to appreciating that each person has a unique and valuable life history. In nursing we have the privilege of being afforded glimpses of our patients' life histories and we share moments in their life journey. In long-term facilities the opportunities to discover and appreciate each person's life story are abundant. Life stories are a way of acknowledging that each individual has a coherent and evolving identity that spans past, present and future.

SOMETHING TO THINK ABOUT

They came
And for a time
They shared
A time, a place, a journey
Anonymous

Reflect on the following 'real-life' stories. Consider how you will practise in a way that acknowledges and respects each individual's personal beliefs, values and needs. Think about how knowing a person's life history may influence your ability to provide person-centred care.

> Megan was a 16-year-old girl with terminal cancer who was admitted to a palliative care unit. All the nursing staff on the unit had become involved in her care, particularly the nurse unit manager. When Megan realised the severity of her condition and that she would not be returning home, she became terribly depressed. The manager spoke to her family and organised a secret 'rendezvous' in the hospital basement, at the service entrance. When Megan was wheeled down to the basement in her hospital bed, surrounded by infusion pumps, syringe drivers and the like, she was greeted by her adored Maltese terrier, Zoe. The look of absolute joy on Megan's face as Zoe snuggled into her arms for the last time was unforgettable.

This caring manager's organisation of a 'rendezvous' was a challenging feat. What elements of this nurse's actions portrayed the true meaning of person-centred care?

> Mrs Trent was in her 80s and admitted for investigation of low haemoglobin levels. A colonoscopy was scheduled, but Mrs Trent was adamant she did not want the procedure. Despite having it explained to her in detail, she refused to consent to it. At times Mrs Trent behaved in a way that indicated she may be confused. For example, she accused a nurse of stealing her purse, which was subsequently found in her drawer. Although she was terribly frightened of the colonoscopy procedure, her son was contacted and he signed the consent for her. The night before the procedure Mrs Trent was supposed to begin drinking several litres of the bowel-preparation solution. At first Mrs Trent refused to drink it, but despite her being distressed, she was eventually coaxed into drinking some of it by a senior nurse. A nursing student stayed with Mrs Trent, with the instruction to 'keep her drinking the solution, until it is all gone. Otherwise the colonoscopy will be a waste of time'.

Was person-centred care evident in this scenario? Carefully consider what you would do if presented with this type of ethical dilemma. (In Chapter 4, we will explore some of the ethical implications of these types of situations more fully.)

Box 1.1   What's in a name?

When describing the people nurses care for, we use the terms 'patient', 'client', 'healthcare consumer' and 'resident'. We made the decision to use these different terms deliberately. When you undertake clinical placements you will quickly become aware that different terms are used to refer to the people you care for, depending on the context of practice (Deber et al. 2005). We define the terms here so you'll have a clear understanding of their meaning.

Box 1.1	*cont'd*

Patient is still the most common term used to describe a person seeking or receiving acute healthcare. It does carry some negative connotations, however, as traditionally a 'patient' was defined as someone who passively endured pain or illness and waited for treatment. Although patients are becoming more active and proactive where their health is concerned, the term 'patient' is still the one you'll hear most often.

Client refers to a recipient of nursing care. 'Client' is a term that is inclusive of individuals, significant others, families and communities. It applies to people who are well and those who are experiencing health changes. It is intended to recognise the recipient of care as an active partner in that care and the need for the nurse to engage in professional behaviours that facilitate this active partnership. The term 'client' is often used in mental health and community health services.

Resident most often refers to a person who resides in a high- or low-care aged care facility or a person with a developmental disability who lives in a residential care facility, either short or long term.

Healthcare consumer is considered by some to be a politically correct term, particularly in the age of consumerism. Some writers (e.g. McLaughlin 2009) suggest that the terms 'patient' and 'client' deny the health-service user the rightful participation that is now expected in the Australian healthcare system. Iedema et al. (2008) identify the healthcare consumer as a co-producer of health, involved in decision making and designing their own care. However, it is important to note that many people deliberately avoid the use of the word 'consumer', claiming that this term is a negative and rather narrow definition of human beings in relationship to sickness and health.

As you can see there are divided opinions about the 'correct' terms to describe the people nurses care for so it is best to keep an open mind during your clinical placements.

SOMETHING TO THINK ABOUT

We would like to challenge you to begin to conceptualise your nursing care as person-centred. For example, what would person-centred pain management look like? How could you administer medications in a person-centred way? What difference would a person-centred approach to hand hygiene make? What is person-centred communication when caring for a person with dementia?

MODELS OF CARE

Undertaking clinical placements in different facilities and units will provide you with exposure to different models of patient care. A model of care provides an approach to the way that patient care is organised within a clinical unit and relates to the way that nurses and other healthcare workers within the team structure patient-care activities. Models of care have evolved over time and continue to receive considerable attention in relation to patient safety and quality (Carlyle et al. 2012; Chiarella & Lau 2007). Historically nursing work was arranged in a hierarchical manner with a charge nurse coordinating and delegating ward work to those below her. Today differences in the models of care implemented within units or wards can be attributed to several factors, including staffing shortages and skill mix (numbers, types and levels of experience of nurses and healthcare workers) (Duffield et al. 2010). Models of patient care may include:

- task-oriented nursing
- team nursing
- patient allocation (or total patient care) (NSW Department of Health 2006; Duffield et al. 2010).

Task-oriented nursing refers to a model in which nurses undertake specific tasks related to nursing care for a group of patients. Some examples of task allocation may be when a nurse showers all or most of the patients in a ward while another nurse administers the medications for the same group of patients. In this model, nursing care relates to sets of activities that are performed by nurses for patients.

Team nursing is a model where experienced nurses are teamed with less experienced or casual staff to achieve nursing goals. The size and skill mix of teams can vary from unit to unit and across healthcare facilities; for example, an experienced registered nurse (RN) may lead a team that consists of a new graduate RN, an endorsed enrolled nurse (EEN) and an assistant in nursing (AIN).

Patient allocation models were developed because nurses recognised the need for total patient care. The implementation of these types of models results in nurses caring for the whole patient rather than focusing on a series of tasks. A nurse will be allocated to his or her patients (the number is dependent on factors such as patient need, staff mix and ward policies) to undertake all nursing care for these allocated patients.

The model of care delivery implemented on a ward depends on a range of factors, including the degree of innovation and commitment by the people involved. Some models work better when there are sufficient numbers of highly qualified staff, such as RNs, to deliver care; others may focus on supporting less experienced staff by using a team approach.

SOMETHING TO THINK ABOUT

On your next placement, identify the model of care delivery used in the unit. Discuss with the nurses the reasons for implementing this model and its advantages and disadvantages. Find out where nursing students, enrolled nurses (ENs) and assistants in nursing (AINs) also fit into this model.

COMPETENT PRACTICE

Competence is a complex concept that is used in various ways in nursing (Garrett et al. 2013). Many people make the mistake of thinking that competence simply means the satisfactory performance of a set task, but competence is much broader than that. The NMBA (2006, p. 10) defines competence as 'The combination of skills, knowledge, attitudes, values and abilities that underpin effective and/or superior performance in a professional/occupational area'.

The attributes and performance required of a competent nurse (or nursing student) are detailed by the NMBA *National competency standards for the registered nurse* (2006). These standards provide a benchmark for assessing competence and are also used in courts of law to determine appropriate professional standards for nursing practice. You will need to become familiar with the competency standards, as your clinical performance will be assessed using these criteria; your eligibility for registration as a nurse will depend on your demonstration of competence. Refer to 'Professional expectations' in Chapter 2 for a more detailed description of the competency standards.

Keep in mind that 'competent' does not mean 'expert' (see Box 1.2). There are various levels of competence, but each has a minimum acceptable standard. Beginners are rarely expert, but they demonstrate safe and effective practice across a range of nursing domains. They may be slow at first and ask many questions (as they should), but they know the right questions to ask.

Box 1.2   What does it all mean?

Competent: The nurse demonstrates competence across all the domains of the competencies applicable to nurses, at a standard that is judged to be appropriate for the level of the nurse being assessed.

Competency standards: These consist of NMBA competency standards that are organised into domains (NMBA 2013). (See Chapter 2 for a more detailed discussion of competency standards.)

Coaching tips

In these coaching tips we suggest ways of developing your competence during your studies and throughout your nursing career.

Be knowledgeable

- Focus on understanding the concepts and principles that underpin nursing care. Knowing why is just as important as knowing how.
- Ask questions and read widely (and constantly).
- Develop your library skills so you can find clinical information fast.
- Develop your research skills so you can discern what is good, better and the best evidence for practice.
- When on a clinical placement, attend educational sessions and inservices whenever you have the opportunity.
- Find out when conferences are being held that are relevant to your learning and attend if possible—they are a great way of networking and accessing cutting-edge information.
- Aim high in your academic pursuits—don't be content with 'just a pass'.

Coaching tips (cont'd)

- Attend all scheduled learning activities.
- Commit to becoming a self-directed, lifelong learner. Remember, 'knowledge keeps no better than fish'; and given the rapid scientific and technological advances in healthcare, the knowledge gained in your program of study may soon become obsolete.

Develop your skills

- Work hard to develop your skills—attend all clinical skills sessions and simulation experiences and actively participate.
- Don't miss an opportunity to practise. Many educational institutions encourage students to practise outside scheduled classes. These are valuable opportunities to consolidate your skills and identify any weaknesses.
- Observe expert clinicians caring for their patients. Ask them to supervise and critique your practice.
- Many types of clinical skill checklists are available and are excellent for assessment purposes. Students can peer-review each other and your clinical educator may use them to assess you. In some programs the assessment of core skills using a designated checklist is a compulsory requirement.
- Continually ask yourself: 'Is my practice safe and effective, and am I adhering to the principles of best practice?'

Learn to think like a nurse

- Nursing is a process of personal and professional growth. Throughout your studies, and indeed your career, it is vitally important to consider and reconsider your values, attitudes and beliefs, and to analyse how these attributes are reflected in your behaviours.
- Reflect on what it is that you value most—in yourself and in other professionals. Is it honesty, integrity, work ethic, compassion? Then consider how these values can be developed and integrated into your practice.
- Challenge your preconceptions, biases, assumptions and prejudices. Listen and be open to other people's perspectives, particularly if their opinions are different from yours.
- Immerse yourself in a wide range of literature and media that challenges your thinking and the way you view the world (there are few worse criticisms for a nurse than to be called narrow-minded or bigoted).
- Embrace cultural diversity and open your mind (and heart) to people of different ethnicity, nationality, religion, language, age and lifestyle—listen and learn!
- Work hard to develop your critical thinking and clinical reasoning abilities (refer to Chapter 4 for more information about these important professional attributes).

WORKING WITHIN YOUR SCOPE OF PRACTICE

'Scope of practice' is a common term in nursing; however, it is not always clearly defined. In this section we refer to scope of practice as the roles, functions, responsibilities, activities and decision-making capacity that nurses (or nursing students) are educated, competent and authorised to perform. A nurse's scope of practice is influenced by the specific setting, legislation, policy, education, standards and the health needs of the population. In Australia the NMBA has emphasised the professional responsibility of:

- understanding one's own scope of practice
- speaking out when an activity is beyond one's scope of practice
- ensuring familiarity with the scope of practice of other healthcare providers to whom one plans to delegate clinical activities or make referrals (NMBA 2007).

Nursing programs differ significantly, so students' scopes of practice will vary depending on where they are enrolled. Your scope of practice will develop as you progress through your nursing program and as your level of competence increases, and it may vary depending on the context of your placement.

Why is it essential to understand and work within your scope of practice?

A scope of practice framework provides parameters that guide clinical learning and the nursing activities that you can participate in. It is not meant to unnecessarily limit your learning but provides a clear outline of the types of activities you should focus on. Consider the following situation:

A first-year student was concerned and upset about his unsatisfactory clinical appraisal. He felt discouraged because he was a high-achieving student who expected to receive an excellent appraisal. The educator had written the following comment: 'Ahmed is a hardworking and committed student but needs to work within his scope of practice and focus on consolidating skills appropriate to his level of enrolment.'

Ahmed complained to his lecturer at university, and she asked him to describe his clinical placement and what had prompted this comment from the educator. Ahmed explained that his placement was great because he had been given wonderful learning opportunities by the doctors and nurses on his ward. He'd been permitted to do central line dressings, titrate IV infusions, manage patient-controlled analgesia (PCA) and more. He was proud that he had learnt skills well beyond those of most first-year students and was annoyed that the educator did not applaud his initiative.

Ahmed had focused on advanced and complex skills without having the necessary theoretical background. Ahmed had not learnt about central lines, infusion pumps or PCAs at university and had little understanding of their purpose or potential complications. Just as worrying was that Ahmed had been so focused on these advanced skills that he'd had little time to practise and consolidate the skills appropriate to his level of enrolment. He was not confident with patient hygiene or vital signs, nor was he able to administer oral medications safely.

Because Ahmed had practised nursing skills outside of his scope of practice, he was considered unsafe. This resulted in a 'fail grade' for his clinical placement. While a scope of practice is not meant to limit learning opportunities, it provides a clear and structured framework for practice, inclusive of your accountability and responsibility. It is developed sequentially so that each new skill is related to and builds on those previously learnt. Most importantly, a scope of practice is supported by related theoretical foundations.

Why do you need to discuss your scope of practice with the nurses you work with?

Clinicians sometimes express the concern that they are not clear about what students have learnt on campus and in previous clinical placements. Additionally, they are unsure of what clinical activities students are permitted to do and should be encouraged to engage in during placements. Clinicians sometimes describe instances where students attempt procedural skills beyond their level of ability or, alternatively, are reluctant to engage in clinical experiences outside of their 'comfort zone'. A clear outline of a student's scope of practice specific to each year of the program allows clinicians to support and challenge students based upon a collaborative understanding of expectations.

Coaching tips

- Make sure you access and understand the scope of practice appropriate to the year of enrolment for your program.
- Clarify how your university requires the scope of practice to be used. Some educational institutions will not permit you to attempt any nursing procedures (a) that are not listed on the scope of practice document, (b) that you have not practised or (c) in which you have not demonstrated competency. Not all programs have the same requirements.
- Share your scope of practice with the nurses you work with so they know how they can best support and guide you.
- Use your scope of practice if you feel pressured to engage in nursing activities that are beyond your level of experience. Simply explain that your institution has parameters that guide your clinical learning but that instead you'd like to watch the procedure being performed by an experienced nurse.
- Remember that a nursing student's scope of practice is not the same as that of an AIN. When you are undertaking a clinical placement you must work within your student scope of practice and if you are working as an AIN you must comply with that specific scope of practice.

SUPERVISION AND SUPPORT

Various models of supporting students' learning are used during clinical placements. The model implemented depends upon various factors, such as the context, the number of students and the student's level of experience. You may have a clinical educator (sometimes called a facilitator) to guide your learning and support you; and/or you may also have the support of an academic visiting the clinical site. You will also have 'mentored' or 'preceptored' placements, in which you are guided by a clinician from the health facility. Depending on the organisational structure of the unit and its staffing levels, you may work with the same RN for the whole placement or you may work with a different nurse every day. There are advantages to both models. Working with the same nurse provides a measure of security and continuity, but you are exposed to only one way of practising. When you work with different nurses you'll experience a range of different practices and this will help clarify the type of nurse you want to be. You will also be challenged to explain and justify your learning objectives more often.

Before your placement, find out the type of support that will be available for you, and ensure you plan learning and assessment activities with this support in mind. Regardless of the type of support provided during placement, it is important to remember that, to a large extent, the success of your placement will depend on what you bring to it and your degree of preparation and motivation.

Your feelings before, during and after your clinical placement experience will vary. Students report experiencing some or all of the following emotions: excitement, exhilaration, pride, confusion, anxiety, fear, apprehension, tension and stress. Your educator or mentor (or both) is there to support you (see Box 1.3). It is important to share your feelings and

Box 1.3 Who shall I turn to?

In Australia and New Zealand, the terms 'mentoring' and 'preceptoring' have evolved and are often used interchangeably to describe a supportive educative role. Mentorship and preceptorship have been described as the most common forms of clinical supervision and support. Both types of supportive relationships have the potential to ease the transition between the relatively sheltered world of academia and the health-service environment.

Mentor: Traditionally, mentoring referred to a mutual and committed relationship between a student or new employee and an experienced staff member. The relationship developed over time and created opportunities for students or new employees to gain valuable skills and knowledge, to become socialised and acculturated to the organisation and its ways of operating and to become proficient under the direct guidance of the mentor.

Preceptor: This term most often refers to a person who orientates students and/or new employees and supports their learning in a designated area, usually over a short period of time. The preceptor acts as a role model and resource person, helping with the process of socialisation.

Buddy: The forces in contemporary practice, such as staffing shortages and increased casualisation of the workforce, sometimes work against sustained, ongoing supportive relationships of mentoring and preceptoring. 'Buddy' is a term that has come to mean a nurse who you work with on a day-by-day basis but not necessarily for an extended period of time.

Practice partner: This more contemporary term refers to a nurse who you work with, often in the final year or semester of your nursing program, who guides and supports you to become increasingly independent, competent, autonomous and responsible.

Clinical educator/facilitator: These staff members may be employed by universities on a casual basis or be seconded from the clinical facilities. Clinical educators assist and enable students in a clinical setting to acquire the required knowledge, skills and attitudes to meet the standards defined by the university and nurse regulatory authorities. Clinical educators liaise between students and academic and clinical staff in a tripartite relationship and are responsible for supporting, teaching and assessing groups of students, often across different wards or units.

Based on Andrews & Roberts (2003); Clare et al. (2002, 2003); Hughes (2002).

SOMETHING TO THINK ABOUT

Mentors remind us that we can indeed survive the terror of the coming journey and undergo the transformation by moving through, not around, our fear. Mentors give us the magic that allows us to enter the darkness, a talisman to protect us from evil spells, a gem of wise advice, a map, and sometimes simply courage. But always the mentor appears near the onset of the journey as a helper, equipping us in some way for what is to come, a midwife to our dreams, a 'keeper of the promise'. Success is a lot more slippery without a mentor to show us the ropes. The mentor is clearly concerned with the transmission of wisdom. They do this by leading us on the journey of our lives. We trust them because they have been there before. They embody our hopes, cast light on the way ahead, interpret arcane signs, warn us of lurking dangers, and point out unexpected delights along the way.

Sources: Daloz 1999 and Parkes 1986

Coaching tips

Irrespective of whether you are supported by a mentor, preceptor, buddy, practice partner or clinical educator, to a large extent the success of the relationship will depend on you. You need to be very clear about your learning objectives (see Chapter 3), as these will frame your learning, and you must be able to explain and elaborate on them so that the person you are working with can support you and guide you towards achieving them. Occasionally, your support person may suggest that your objectives need to be modified or amended if they are not achievable or appropriate for a particular environment.

You need to be able to define your scope of practice so that your support person is aware of what you can and can't do. You will probably find that your mentor/preceptor will observe and assess you for a while before entrusting you with patient care. Don't take this personally or as an indication of a lack of confidence in your ability. It is to be expected. RNs maintain responsibility for their patients at all times and so need to be very sure of your abilities before allowing you to practise with any measure of independence. The degree of supervision provided to you will vary with your level of experience and the degree of patient acuity.

If a situation arises in which you feel that your relationship with your support person is not working, try to resolve it with them in the first instance. Be open to their viewpoints, as it may just be a problem of miscommunication. However, if this does not improve

Coaching tips (cont'd)

the situation or if you feel uncomfortable about trying to resolve it, you should seek the support and guidance of someone experienced who you feel you can trust to handle the situation professionally—your facilitator or academic staff, for example.

Nursing mirrors what happens in everyday life and sometimes personality clashes arise. Hopefully, these can be managed in a positive, professional and constructive manner, but at times it may be best for you to work with a different person. Be mindful that experiencing a series of personality clashes may indicate that you need some guidance in managing interpersonal relationships.

STUDENT STORY
If you get a good mentor you know you're set. That connection is the key.
Emma's story

In this story Emma, a third-year nursing student, describes how consistent, quality mentorship facilitated a sense of belonging and helped her to fit into the clinical environment. She recalls how her developing relationship with her mentor promoted her learning, enhanced her confidence and challenged her thinking.

If you get a good mentor you know you're set. That connection is the key to fitting into the ward, and one person can make all the difference. On my last placement I was with the same mentor for almost two weeks. That made a huge difference. She knew where I was at ... she knew what I wanted to get out of the placement because we'd already discussed it, so we didn't need to talk about it again. I was really proactive because I had a lot that I wanted to get out of the two weeks and I knew I was going to be pushing time. So I was very clear about sitting down with her and showing her my objectives very early on. She also knew where my skills were at after the first couple of days of watching me and helping me. That makes such a big difference to what happened in that two weeks. Because she wasn't constantly assessing me, like when you've got a different RN every day. They assess you for the first half of it before they'll let you have that little bit more leeway, or encourage you to take a few more steps towards developing skills and things. So by the end of the first week she knew exactly what I could and couldn't do competently, and how much she could push me. She knew what she had to educate me on and what she didn't have to educate me on.

It really felt great because when you have to go through that every day you don't feel like you're getting anywhere. You feel like you're repeating the same stuff all the time. I felt like she was enabling me to really consolidate all the skills I already had and extend them. I felt like I had the power to turn around and say, 'I know how to do that, do you mind if I go and have a look at that because I haven't done that before, or I haven't seen that before?'

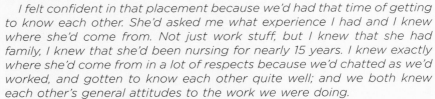

STUDENT STORY *cont'd*

I felt confident in that placement because we'd had that time of getting to know each other. She'd asked me what experience I had and I knew where she'd come from. Not just work stuff, but I knew that she had family, I knew that she'd been nursing for nearly 15 years. I knew exactly where she'd come from in a lot of respects because we'd chatted as we'd worked, and gotten to know each other quite well; and we both knew each other's general attitudes to the work we were doing.

We didn't always have similar attitudes, but we could see each other's points of view because we'd been able to chat around it, and I think in a lot of ways we had a very similar outlook. Just because we don't necessarily agree with everything that somebody else tells us doesn't mean that it's not valid either. So we both had that sort of point of view where we're quite open to other people's opinions ... without necessarily having to agree with them.

Remember: Think about the actions taken by Emma that made this mentor–mentee relationship such a positive experience. Which of these could you emulate on your next clinical placement?

Source: Levett-Jones et al. 2007

to seek further guidance and support whenever necessary. During and/or at the conclusion of your placement your educator will also provide you with opportunities for debriefing, reflection, discussion and learning from your clinical experiences.

Student support services

There may be times before, during or following your clinical placements when you need additional guidance or support. Support services are available at your educational institution and many healthcare facilities also provide these services.

Table 1.1 lists some of the support mechanisms that may be available. Be proactive in identifying supports early in your student life. It is easier to access and use services if you know about them in advance, rather than to start from scratch when you have a problem.

Table 1.1 Where to find support during clinical placement

Type of support	Services available
Academic	• Learning workshops associated with mathematics and drug calculations • Writing assistance • Peer mentoring (e.g. for nursing skill development or feedback on skill performance) • Online resources (e.g. <www.metamath.com/multiple/multiple_choice_questions.html> or <www.engr.ncsu.edu/learningstyles/ilsweb.html>)

Table 1.1 *cont'd*

Type of support	Services available
Accommodation	Available through some healthcare institutions (ask your clinical coordinator or check the institution's website)
Advocacy	• Clinical educators • Mentors • Lecturers or other staff at the educational institution • Clinical coordinator (education- or facility-based) • Student bodies, associations • Professional organisations (e.g. nursing colleges), dean of students, student union
Chaplains	Discussion of experiences and feelings from clinical or pastoral care
Counselling services	• Personal development (e.g. how to get along with difficult people or how to gain insight into your own behaviour) • Discussion of clinical issues (e.g. caring for a person who is dying) • Stress-management strategies • Time-management strategies
Disability advisors	Resources and avenues for assistance such as assessments for fitness to practice. Registration for this service is required in most educational institutions
General practitioners, emergency departments	Medical assistance associated with clinical placement including: • immunisations before entry into a health facility • advice about medical problems before a placement • medical clearance before a placement • treatment for a needle-stick injury • other injury during placement
Language (students from non-English-speaking backgrounds)	Advice available from: • the international unit at your educational institution • the learning support unit
Scholarships	• International exchange to experience a placement overseas • Fee support • Workplace scholarships • Fee support for a clinical placement • State or territory health department • Nursing scholarship, aged care scholarships or assistance to attend special placements (e.g. rural placements) For details see websites of your university, healthcare institution, state/territory government, registration board, professional groups and associations
Policy breach assistance (e.g. harassment, bullying, privacy issues)	As for advocacy

SOMETHING TO THINK ABOUT

Investigate the student support services that are available at your educational and healthcare institutions. Identify how these services can be of support to you before, during or after your clinical placement.

WORKING HARD TO BELONG

Nursing students frequently express how important it is for them to fit in—to belong and be accepted as part of the nursing team (Levett-Jones & Lathlean 2009). This is not surprising given that the need to belong has long been cited as a fundamental human need (Baumeister & Leary 1995; Maslow 1987). Students who try too hard to fit in sometimes sacrifice their 'student status' to become one of the 'workers'. It is not unusual for students, believing that their hard work will help them to be valued as part of the team, to fill their clinical placement days with a series of disjointed nursing tasks (making beds, taking vital signs, bathing patients) rather than developing their ability to nurse holistically. Don't be confused! Students should certainly practise nursing skills. However, as a student you need to be proactive in identifying and maximising valuable learning opportunities across a range of areas and at different levels.

Coaching tips

Give yourself permission to be a student! Explain your learning objectives and assessment requirements. Be on the lookout for serendipitous learning opportunities. Listen closely to your educator and mentor in handover and relate your clinical objectives to the clinical issues identified; for example, if someone mentions a complex diabetic leg ulcer that needs to be re-dressed and you have wound management as one of your objectives, take the initiative! Ask if you can watch the wound dressing being performed, then research all you can about diabetic ulcers. The next day ask if you can undertake the procedure under supervision. As a student it is your responsibility to link theory and practice and you will have countless opportunities to do so (if you are on the lookout for them). Linking theory to practice will allow you to develop your repertoire of knowledge and skills in a way that is clinically relevant.

Ask if you can care for increasing numbers of patients (under supervision) so you can develop your time-management and organisational skills (even in your first year). While caring for groups of patients you'll be practising nursing skills (never forget how important they are and how much consolidation they need), but you'll also be extending your practice and learning to nurse holistically rather than in a task-oriented way.

Don't think that if you just 'get on with the job' you'll fit in and be accepted. You are much more likely to earn the respect of your colleagues by fully embracing your student status, asking questions, seeking learning opportunities and showing an interest.

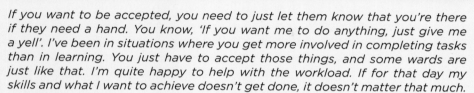

STUDENT STORY

Working hard for acceptance
Laura's story

If you want to be accepted, you need to just let them know that you're there if they need a hand. You know, 'If you want me to do anything, just give me a yell'. I've been in situations where you get more involved in completing tasks than in learning. You just have to accept those things, and some wards are just like that. I'm quite happy to help with the workload. If for that day my skills and what I want to achieve doesn't get done, it doesn't matter that much.

Critically reflect on Laura's story and contemplate what it might mean for her learning experience (or yours if you were to take her advice).

Source: Levett-Jones et al. 2007

FIRST IMPRESSIONS LAST

It's sad but true that first impressions are formed within seconds of meeting, and such impressions are based most often on appearance. The opinions of clinicians and patients will be influenced as much by your professional appearance (or lack of) as by your actual performance. Forget what you see on television. In the real world of nursing, a very specific dress code exists. The clinical environment is focused on safety—yours and that of the patients—and this, to a large extent, dictates what is considered acceptable in appearances in general, and in uniforms in particular.

Don't be caught unaware—before you begin your placement, check your educational institution's requirements as well as those of your placement venue. Some students may require modifications to be made to their uniform for a variety of reasons. Head scarfs etc. worn for cultural or religious reasons are usually expected to be the same colour as your uniform. If you need to wear long sleeves they will need to be loose enough to be pulled up (and not slip down) when undertaking hand hygiene and nursing procedures. In addition, some placements have special requirements; for example, mental health facilities may prefer smart casual clothes, while operating theatres provide surgical attire.

Below we offer some guidelines based on our experiences of what most clinical venues expect. We tried to find a way of writing this section that was discreet and delicate but eventually decided to just 'say it like it is'!

Coaching tips

- Uniforms should be neat, complete, correctly fitting, freshly washed and ironed for each shift.

- Shoes must be comfortable (for obvious reasons) and comply with workplace health and safety standards (non-slip, fully enclosed, leather). Runners are great for sport, but not for a clinical placement.

- Heavy makeup is not appropriate for clinical placements. Overpowering perfumes should be avoided as they can cause patients to become nauseated.

Coaching tips

Coaching tips (cont'd)

- Nails should be clean, short, filed and without nail polish for infection-control purposes. It is easy to tear the fragile skins of elderly patients or penetrate gloves with long or sharp nails. Chipped nail polish and artificial nails harbour infectious microorganisms.

- Long hair must be clean and tied back firmly.

- For men, beards should be neat and trimmed.

- Leave your jewellery at home. Wristwatches are problematic because they can scratch patients and need to be removed each time you wash your hands. A fob watch is more convenient. Similarly, rings can scratch patients and cause cross-infection. A plain band is usually acceptable in most clinical areas. Remove body piercings. One pair of small studs (in ears only) may be accepted, but bracelet(s) or necklace(s) are not to be worn (unless of the medic alert type). Many confused patients have pulled or grabbed at a dangling necklace or earring (ouch!).

- For those placements where smart casual clothing is requested in lieu of uniform, avoid wearing revealing clothing. A corporate approach is usually expected.

  It may not be polite to mention the following issues in refined company, but ...

  - Please shower/bathe daily (and wear deodorant).

  - There is nothing worse for a nauseated patient than being cared for by a nurse who smells of cigarette smoke or who has bad breath. Clean teeth and fresh breath are essential.

- Last, but not least, make sure you always wear your official university ID or name badge and have your personal protective equipment (e.g. safety glasses) with you on clinical placements.

MANDATORY REQUIREMENTS FOR CLINICAL PLACEMENTS

In order for students to undertake placements, several requirements are dictated by governing bodies before students can enter a healthcare facility. These requirements are based on a duty of care to vulnerable clients and a commitment to minimising risk (both to patients and to you). You are responsible for providing evidence of complying with these requirements either to a member of staff from the healthcare facility or at compliance screening sessions undertaken on campus pre-placement. Failure to provide complete documentary evidence of meeting the mandatory requirements will usually mean you are not allocated a clinical placement or that your placement is cancelled. Evidence you will be required to produce can include vaccination cards, related medical reports (such as serology tests) and a national police check. Any documented criminal recordings will require you to undertake a risk assessment before placement is allocated.

The requirements for entry into a healthcare facility vary across Australia and New Zealand and may be different depending on the type of healthcare organisation where you undertake your placement (e.g. public and private facilities, aged care facilities, hospitals or education facilities). For advice about mandatory requirements you should check your university policies and protocols well in advance of placement as requirements may take several weeks or even months to be finalised. Government health websites also provide this information in the form of policy statements for employment or clinical placements.

Examples of mandatory requirements required for placements may include:

- prohibited employment declaration
- working with children check
- aged care check
- police check
- occupational assessment, screening and vaccinations against specified infectious diseases.

In addition to mandatory requirements you also have a responsibility to ensure you are fit for practice. Issues such as serious long-term physical or mental health conditions (including substance abuse) or professional misconduct that might impair your ability to undertake clinical placements must be declared and discussed with the appropriate person at your educational institution so that realistic support and advice can be provided.

Coaching tips

- Complete all checks as soon as practical after enrolment in your degree or diploma.
- Be aware that your placement will be cancelled if you do not comply with the mandatory requirements by a specified date.
- Undertake vaccinations as per the health schedule early in the program, and provide serology for proof of immunisation as required.
- Ensure you have all of the required information with you when you are on a clinical placement—information may be called upon at any time.
- Always keep mandatory requirements information in a safe place because you may need it for each new placement and upon application for future nursing positions.
- If you lose your mandatory requirements information, immediately take steps to obtain replacements.
- Keep a copy of your information to make it easier to secure replacement cards/reports.
- Report changes to your criminal record as necessary—see government policy information for clarification.

THE ROLES AND RESPONSIBILITIES OF THE INTERPROFESSIONAL HEALTHCARE TEAM

Up until this section our discussion has been predominantly nursing-focused. However, safe healthcare delivery requires a broader approach. Effective clinical care depends upon each member of the interprofessional team knowing and understanding the roles and responsibilities of the others. However, too often this is not the case. In a recent research project nursing, pharmacy and medical graduates were interviewed about their understanding of the roles of members of the healthcare team. Their insights highlighted the nature and extent of the problem:

> The [interprofessional] healthcare team comes up in every single lecture but not what a doctor's role is, or what a nurse's role is. We come into the workforce, not really knowing what they do, or what they know, or how to talk to them—Pharmacy graduate.
>
> (Levett-Jones et al. 2014)

A medical graduate, when discussing his lack of familiarity with the roles of the members of the healthcare team, said:

> It's almost like a tradesman having a toolbox that they've never opened, and every now and again somebody tells them that there's a tool that could be useful, might make a certain job easier ... but if you don't know about it, you can't use it.
>
> (Levett-Jones et al. 2014)

Similarly a nursing graduate commented:

> I think a lot of doctors don't actually have a clue what nurses do. I mean they write orders, they get followed through, and as long as they get followed through, they [the doctors] don't really notice what else we do. So they don't know how we assess patients and they don't trust our examinations.
>
> (Levett-Jones et al. 2014)

These graduates' comments emphasise the importance of learning about the other members of the healthcare team. There is clear evidence that you cannot communicate and collaborate effectively with other members of the healthcare team unless you understand, respect and value each person's role. Aside from nurses, the healthcare team may include medical and allied health personnel such as pharmacists, physiotherapists, pathologists, psychologists, counsellors, radiologists, occupational therapists and speech pathologists, to name a few. Table 1.2 provides a brief outline of the roles of a number of the members of the interprofessional healthcare team. In Chapter 5 we will turn our attention to how the members of interprofessional team communicate for the benefit of patients.

Table 1.2 Members of the interprofessional healthcare team

Role	Definition
Student—nursing or midwifery	People who are enrolled in educational programs accredited by registration boards that authorise nursing and midwifery. These may include undergraduate nurses, enrolled nurses and student midwives.

Table 1.2 *cont'd*

Role	Definition
Registered nurse (RN)	A person whose name is entered on the register allocated to RNs. RNs are responsible and accountable for providing nursing care to patients.
Enrolled nurse	A person whose name is entered on the register allocated to enrolled nurses. Enrolled nurses practise under the direction of an RN. An extension of the category of enrolled nurse (e.g. endorsed enrolled nurse) is a person who performs at an advanced level and is delegated higher responsibilities (such as medication administration) under the supervision of an RN or a midwife.
Midwife	A person whose name is entered in the register for practice. Qualifications and experience are approved by the registering authority, to render the person capable of providing maternity services to mothers and babies.
Nurse practitioner	An RN or midwife who has been educated to function autonomously and collaboratively in an advanced and extended role and whose scope of practice is determined by his or her context of practice.
Healthcare worker	Various roles are undertaken by healthcare workers. They may function independently or in collaboration with the interdisciplinary healthcare team. Examples would be an Aboriginal or Maori healthcare worker, physio assistant and dietary assistant. Some roles may be accountable to the RN or midwife.
Unregulated carer	A variety of roles exist for people who care for patients without licensing requirements. They may undertake activities delegated by the RN or midwife according to their competence. Examples are carers, personal care assistants and AINs.
Patient care attendant	People employed by a facility to support the care requirements of patients. They may have functions that involve moving or positioning patients and/or equipment, attending to the personal needs of patients or disposing of soiled equipment. Functions associated with this position are varied and often depend on the context of the area in which they are employed.
Technician	Various technical positions abound in healthcare facilities. Some of these have replaced nursing roles and others have supplementary roles in the care of clients. Examples of technical staff are technicians who work with specialist equipment—for example, anaesthetic technicians and sterile-supply technicians.

Table 1.2 *cont'd*

Role	Definition
Medical personnel	You will encounter several levels of medical personnel during placement. Public healthcare facilities employ resident medical officers, whereas other institutions may use the consultancy services of medical officers. This will depend on the nature of the facility (i.e. public or private) and the agreements in place between the facility and medical officer. Resident medical officers usually encountered in public hospitals include: • intern • resident medical officer (year 1–4) • registrar (year 1–4) • senior registrar. Consultant medical officers may have the following positions: anaesthetists, surgeons, obstetricians, gynaecologists, physicians, pathologists, psychiatrists, etc.
Pharmacist	Nurses interact with pharmacists in healthcare in varying ways but especially in regard to dispensing safe and appropriate medication. A pharmacist is a health professional with the knowledge and skills to educate patients about the use of medications to achieve optimal health outcomes. A pharmacist undertakes a university program in pharmacy and is required to be registered.
Social worker	Social workers provide support to clients by dealing with social, emotional and environmental problems associated with an illness, a disability or hospitalisation. Social workers have usually undertaken an advanced education and may specialise in areas such as medical social work (to support patients and their families in hospital settings) or psychiatric social work if they have specialised in counselling patients and their families in dealing with social, emotional or environmental problems relating to mental illness.
Dietician	A dietician is a university-qualified expert in nutrition and dietetics who applies the science of nutritional principles to the planning and preparation of foods and regulation in the diet. They provide dietetic services using best-practice guidelines to promote optimal nutritional status and self-management of disease. Dieticians also participate in health promotion and community health projects.
Psychologist	A person who is engaged in the scientific study of the mind and behaviour, and may provide clinical treatment and teaching. They may be concerned with different areas, such as sport and exercise, education and occupational or clinical psychology.
Podiatrist	A practitioner of podiatry (chiropody) who deals with the conditions of feet and their ailments.

Table 1.2 *cont'd*

Role	Definition
Occupational therapist	A person who employs a form of therapy for those recuperating from physical or mental disease or injury. They encourage rehabilitation through performance of the activities of daily living (such as washing and dressing, hobbies and work).
Speech pathologist	A person concerned with the study and treatment of clients with speech, communication, language and swallowing problems.
Counsellor	A person who supports clients to deal with personal problems that do not involve psychological disorders.
Physiotherapist	A physiotherapist treats congenital and movement disorders across the life span through: education; retraining of movement patterns; specific exercises for improving strength; endurance; flexibility and motor control; and joint and soft-tissue mobilisation. They might also use electrophysical modalities.

Based on Baron & Kalsher (2002); *Concise Medical Dictionary* (Oxford Reference Online); NSW Department of Health (2007); Nurses Board of Western Australia (2004); National Health Workforce Taskforce (2009); ANMC and Nursing Council of New Zealand (2010); Harris et al. (2010).

Coaching tips

A practical and accurate understanding of the role of each member of the interprofessional healthcare team can only be achieved through observation and asking questions. When on clinical placements seek opportunities to observe and communicate with members of the team about their roles, responsibilities and values. This knowledge will be invaluable in helping you to communicate effectively and work collaboratively to promote patient safety and wellbeing.

References

Andrews M, Roberts D. Supporting student nurses learning in and through clinical practice: the role of the clinical guide. *Nurse Educ Today*. 2003;23:474-481.

ANMC. *ANMC National Competency Standards for the Registered Nurse*. Canberra: Australian Nursing and Midwifery Council; 2006.

Baron RA, Kalsher MJ. *Essentials of Psychology*. Boston: Allyn and Bacon; 2002.

Bauman A, Fardy H, Harris P. Getting it right: why bother with patient-centred care? *Med J Aust*. 2003;179: 253-256.

Baumeister R, Leary M. The need to belong: desire for interpersonal attachments as a fundamental human motivation. *Psychol Bull*. 1995;117(3):497-529.

Carlyle D, Crowe M, Deering D. Models of care delivery in mental health nursing practice: a mixed method study. *J Psychiatr Ment Health Nurs*. 2012;19(3):221-230.

Chiarella M, Lau C. *Second report on the models of care project: workshops and seminars February-December 2006*. Sydney: NSW Health; 2007. Online. Available: <www.health.nsw.gov.au>; Accessed 02.03.14.

Clare J, White J, Edwards H, et al. *Curriculum, clinical education, recruitment, transition and retention in nursing: final report for the AUTC, January*. Adelaide: School of Nursing and Midwifery, Flinders University; 2002.

Clare J, Brown D, Edwards H, et al. *Evaluating clinical learning environments: creating education–practice partnerships and clinical education benchmarks for nursing. Learning outcomes and curriculum development in major disciplines: nursing phase 2 final report, March.* Adelaide: School of Nursing and Midwifery, Flinders University; 2003.

Daloz N. *Guiding the journey of adult learners.* San Francisco: Jossey Bass; 1999.

Deber RB, Kraetschmer N, Urowitz S, et al. Patient, consumer, client, or customer: what do people want to be called? *Health Expect.* 2005;8(4):345-351.

Department of Health and Ageing. *Building a 21st century primary health care system: Australia's first national primary health care strategy.* Canberra: Department of Health and Ageing; 2010. Online. Available: <http://www.yourhealth.gov.au/internet/yourhealth/publishing.nsf/Content/Building-a-21st-Century-Primary-Health-Care-System-TOC#.ULZ0-HolqSo>; Accessed 23.02.14.

Desai RJ, Williams CE, Greene SB, et al. Analysis of medication errors in North Carolina nursing homes. *J Pain Palliat Care.* 2013;27(2):125-131.

Duffield C, Roche M, Diers D, et al. Staffing, skill mix and the model of care. *J Clin Nurs.* 2010; 19(15-16):2242-2251.

Garrett BM, MacPhee M, Jackson C. Evaluation of an eportfolio for the assessment of clinical competence in a baccalaureate nursing program. *Nurse Educ Today.* 2013;33(10):1207-1213.

Harris P, Nagy S, Vardaxis N. *Mosby's Dictionary of Medicine, Nursing & Health Professions.* Sydney: Mosby Elsevier; 2010.

Hughes C. Issues in supervisory facilitation. *Studies in Continuing Education.* 2002;24(1):57-71.

Iedema R, Sorensen R, Jorm C, et al. Co-producing care. In: Sorensen R, Iedema R, eds. *Managing clinical processes in health care.* Sydney: Churchill Livingstone Elsevier; 2008:105-120.

Institute for Patient- and Family-Centered Care. *Advancing the practice of patient- and family-centered care: how to get started.* Bethesda: Institute for Patient- and Family-Centered Care; 2008.

Karavasiliadou S, Athanasakis E. An inside look into the factors contributing to medication errors in the clinical nursing practice. *Health Sci J.* 2014;8(1):32-44.

Levett-Jones T, Gilligan C, Outram S, et al. Key attributes of 'patient safe' communication. In: Levett-Jones T, ed. *Critical conversations for patient safety: an essential guide for health professionals.* Sydney: Pearson; 2014.

Levett-Jones T, Lathlean J. The 'Ascent to Competence' conceptual framework: an outcome of a study of belongingness. *J Clin Nurs.* 2009;18:2870-2879.

Levett-Jones T, Lathlean J, McMillan M, et al. Belongingness: a montage of nursing students' stories of their clinical placement experiences. *Contemporary Nurse.* 2007;24(2):162-174.

Levinson W, Lesser C, Epstein R. Developing physician communication skills for patient-centered care. *Health Aff.* 2010;29(7):1310-1318.

Maslow A. *Motivation and personality.* 3rd ed. New York: Harper and Row; 1987.

McLaughlin H. What's in a name: 'Client', 'patient', 'customer', 'consumer', 'expert by experience', 'service user'—what's next? *Br J Soc Work.* 2009;39(6):1101-1117.

Meterko M, Wright S, Lin H, et al. Mortality among patients with acute myocardial infarction: the influences of patient-centered care and evidence-based medicine. *Health Serv Res.* 2010;45(5 Pt 1):1188-1204.

NSW Department of Health. *First report on the Models of Care Project, February–April 2005.* North Sydney: NSW Department of Health; 2006.

NSW Department of Health. Medical Officers Employment Arrangements in the NSW Public Service System. Online. Available: <www.health.nsw.gov.au/policies/PD2007_087>; 2007 Accessed 30.12.09.

Nurses Board of Western Australia. Scope of Nursing Practice Decision-Making Framework. Online. Available: <www.nmbwa.org.au>; 2004 Accessed 30.12.09.

Nursing and Midwifery Board of Australia (NMBA). *National competency standards for the registered nurse.* Online. Available: <www.nursingmidwiferyboard.gov.au>; 2006 Accessed 23.02.14.

Nursing and Midwifery Board of Australia (NMBA). *Code of professional conduct for nurses in Australia.* Online. Available: <www.nursingmidwiferyboard.gov.au>; 2008 Accessed 23.02.14.

Nursing and Midwifery Board of Australia (NMBA). *A national framework for the development and decision-making tools for nursing and midwifery practice.* Online. Available: <www.nursingmidwiferyboard.gov.au>; 2007 Accessed 23.02.14.

Parkes S. *The critical years: the young adult's search for faith to live by.* San Francisco: Harper; 1986.

Reid-Searl K, Moxham L, Happell B. Enhancing patient safety: the importance of direct supervision for avoiding medication errors and near misses by undergraduate nursing students. *Int J Nurs Pract.* 2010;16(3): 225-232.

Tran DT, Johnson M. Classifying nursing errors in clinical management within an Australian hospital. *Int Nurs Rev.* 2010;57(4):454-462.

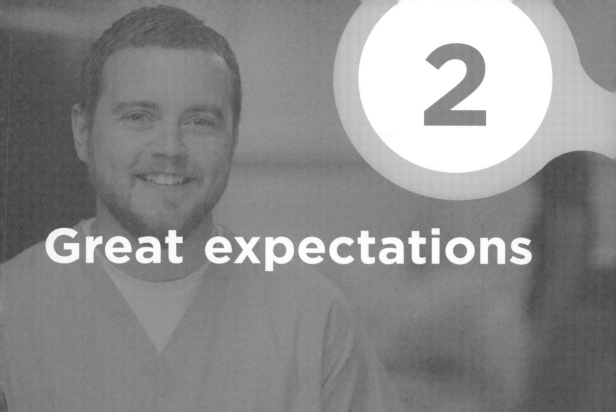

Great expectations

Our environment, the world in which we live and work, is a mirror of our attitudes and expectations.

Earl Nightingale

INTRODUCTION

This chapter provides insights into what you can expect when you undertake clinical placements and what others will expect of you. We consider these issues from different perspectives and describe the expectations of key stakeholders—patients, clinicians, professional organisations and educators. We also discuss legal requirements and your rights and responsibilities as a student.

PATIENTS' EXPECTATIONS

What do patients expect from their nurse? Ask your friends, family and fellow students this question and you are bound to get a wide range of responses. What nursing attributes do you think are most important to patients? Research indicates that caring, empathy, listening, 'being with', comforting and communication are qualities that patients value highly (McCormack et al. 2008). However, the saying 'the patient doesn't care how much you know, they just want to know how much you care' is not completely true. Certainly, patients want to be able to depend on you to take care of them with kindness and empathy, but, with the increasing complexity of healthcare, patients also want to be sure you are knowledgeable and technically capable. For example, a group of women undergoing chemotherapy for cancer were asked what they valued most in the nurses caring for them. They agreed it was essential, first, that the nurses were knowledgeable about and skilled in the management of chemotherapy; and second, that they took the time to demonstrate genuine care and empathy (McIlfatrick et al. 2007).

The Australian Charter of Healthcare Rights (Box 2.1) outlines patients' rights and expectations regarding healthcare provision and emphasises the importance of communication and working in partnership with patients.

Box 2.1	The Australian Charter of Healthcare Rights

Safety: a right to safe and high-quality care

Respect: a right to be shown respect, dignity and consideration

Communication: a right to be informed about services, treatment options and costs in a clear and open way

Participation: a right to be included in decisions and choices about care

Privacy: a right to privacy and confidentiality of provided information

Comment: a right to comment on care and having concerns addressed

Source: Australian Commission on Safety and Quality in Health Care 2012

So what does this mean for nursing students? If patients have high expectations of the people who care for them, how will they respond to being cared for by students? We can assure you that most patients are very supportive of students and will not expect you to perform every procedure perfectly. For example, if you are unsure the first few times when taking a temperature or blood pressure, patients will understand. When you are slow at dressing a wound or removing an intravenous (IV) cannula, patients will make allowances because you are still learning. If you are hesitant or lacking in confidence as a beginning student most people will be patient and encouraging.

There are some things that patients do not make allowances for however, irrespective of the nurse's experience or level. Patients expect nursing students to be as respectful of their privacy and dignity as any other nurse would be. They expect you to be honest about what you know and don't know, and what you can and can't do. They expect you to be courteous and to treat them with respect at all times. Even though you are a learner, patients still expect you to carry out procedures safely and accurately and to acknowledge your limitations and scope of practice. Additionally, while patients will not expect you to be able to answer all their questions, they will expect you to find someone who can.

Patients often comment that they appreciate being cared for by students because they take the time to stop and talk. In busy hospital units this is often undervalued. Many patients also like to feel they have been involved in the clinical education of nursing students and will happily explain their history, diagnosis, treatment regimen and medications. Listen carefully; you will learn a great deal from your patients—they are the experts about their lives and health conditions. Listen to them, learn from them and appreciate their stories. They contain a wealth of information that you can use to plan and implement nursing interventions that are informed by a person-centred approach.

Coaching tips

- Make sure you are prepared before you enter a patient's room. It is very disconcerting for a patient when a student does not understand what they are doing or why they are doing it. If you are giving a subcutaneous injection, for example, review the patient history and the procedure; discuss the details with your mentor, and ask as many questions as necessary, before you approach your patient.

- Admit when you are out of your depth. If an infusion pump is alarming and you don't know how to deal with it, don't pretend you do. Find someone who can assist you (then watch and learn).

- If you are taking blood pressure or performing any other observation, and you are really not sure if your result is correct, be honest and ask someone to check it for you.

- Remember that, while technical competence is essential, nursing should not be reduced to a series of tasks that lack the therapeutic qualities so important to patients.

SOMETHING TO THINK ABOUT

When exploring patients' expectations it is essential to ask their views. In 2009 Australian patients and their families were surveyed in an attempt to clarify what their priorities were when undergoing healthcare. In the list below note how many of the priorities identified relate to effective communication:

- Healthcare professionals discussing anxieties and fears with the patient
- Patients having confidence and trust in healthcare professionals
- The ease of finding someone to talk to about concerns
- Doctors and nurses answering patients' questions understandably
- Patients receiving enough information about their condition and/or treatment
- Test results being explained understandably
- Patients having enough say about and being involved in care and/or treatment decisions
- Being given information about patients' rights and responsibilities
- Staff doing everything possible to control pain

Source: New South Wales Health 2009

CLINICIANS' EXPECTATIONS

Like patients, the clinicians you work with on clinical placements will have realistic expectations of your abilities and level of knowledge. They will understand that you are not an expert and that you are there to learn. Listed below are clinicians' expectations of nursing students that have been consistently identified as important to successful clinical placements. Take some time to think about each of these points.

Students should:

- make an effort to learn about the clinical context and the work they are involved in
- know when to ask questions and where to go for help
- recognise their own limitations and strengths
- demonstrate commitment to the nursing team
- ask questions and question practice
- be critical-thinking problem-solvers
- be positive, motivated and enthusiastic about undertaking a clinical placement
- know their scope of practice and be able to communicate this to their mentor
- become competent at essential nursing skills
- take advantage of all learning opportunities provided
- be open to the suggestions and guidance offered
- develop good interpersonal skills and be friendly and respectful of others
- practise according to workplace health and safety requirements
- understand the importance of accurate documentation and other legal and ethical issues
- come to the clinical placement adequately prepared and with clear and realistic clinical learning objectives.

Do these expectations seem realistic to you? How do you measure up? It is always interesting, and sometimes surprising, to see a situation from another person's perspective. We have spent time with students who were really not aware of what clinicians expected of them and were confused and sometimes dismayed by the feedback they received. When the situation is as important as your clinical placement experience, it is vital that you consider it from many perspectives.

MANAGERS' EXPECTATIONS

It would be nice to think that as students step into a clinical unit, excited and ready to begin their placement, the nursing unit manager will be there, standing at the door, smiling in welcome. Perhaps in the ideal world the manager might compliment students frequently on their skills and make wonderful comments about them to the other staff. You may also think that the manager will understand if you are late for the shift, not in correct uniform, or a little tired or unmotivated. Reality check! Nurse managers are busy people. Their first responsibility is patient welfare. They are responsible for budgets, equipment, resources, standards of practice, workplace health and safety, rostering, staffing issues, quality management, infection control—the list goes on. Students are only one of many important considerations for managers. Consequently they will expect you to meet the same professional standards as their staff in terms of presentation, punctuality, work ethics, standards of practice, etc.

Students sometimes complain when they are reminded by a manager 'not to be late', to 'wear the correct uniform' or to 'tie their hair up', believing that because they are not employees the manager has no authority over them. Students need to be aware that the manager is responsible for all that occurs in the unit and is committed to maintaining professional practice standards. They have the final say on who does (and does not) undertake a placement there. A failure to meet professional standards may jeopardise patient safety and as a result students may be asked to leave the clinical area if they do not meet these expectations.

PROFESSIONAL EXPECTATIONS

In Australia and New Zealand (as in most countries) the professional expectations of nurses are spelled out very clearly. Nurses are required to provide high-quality care through safe and effective clinical practice. National standards and guidelines for registered and enrolled nurses were developed by the Australian Nursing and Midwifery Council (ANMC) and recently became the jurisdiction of the Nursing and Midwifery Board of Australia (NMBA). These standards and guidelines are reviewed regularly to ensure that they reflect contemporary practice. The standards include the:

- *National competency standards for the registered nurse* (2006)
- *National competency standards for the enrolled nurse* (2002)
- *Code of ethics for nurses in Australia* (2008a)
- *Code of professional conduct for nurses in Australia* (2008b).

Likewise, the Nursing Council of New Zealand has a published set of standards and guidelines for nurses. These include:

- *Competencies for registered nurses* (2007)
- *Code of conduct for nurses* (2012)
- *Guidelines for cultural safety, the Treaty of Waitangi and Maori health* (2011).

In addition the New Zealand Nurses Organisation has published its *Code of ethics* (2010).

These standards, codes and guidelines communicate to the general public, particularly healthcare consumers, the knowledge, skills, behaviours, attitudes and values expected of nurses. We encourage you to become familiar with these codes and standards as they are the professional expectations that form the framework against which your practice will be assessed. You will be required to demonstrate that you have met these standards as an indication that you are fit to provide safe, competent care in a variety of settings. Your ability to meet these standards will determine your eligibility for registration and your ability to maintain your registration as a practising nurse. Throughout this book you will see that we often refer to the NMBA and Nursing Council of New Zealand codes and standards in order to help you become familiar with their use and application in practice.

National competency standards for nurses

The *National competency standards for the registered nurse* are an Australian benchmark for registered nurses, and they reinforce responsibility and accountability in delivering quality nursing care through safe and effective practice. These standards are also used in courts of law to determine appropriate professional standards for nursing practice. The competency standards are organised into four domains:

1. **Professional practice:** This relates to the professional, legal and ethical responsibilities that require demonstration of a satisfactory knowledge base, accountability for practice, functioning in accordance with legislation that affects nursing and healthcare, and the protection of individual and group rights.

2. **Critical thinking and analysis:** This relates to self-appraisal, professional development and the value of evidence and research for practice. The ability to engage in reflective practice is also considered an important professional benchmark.

3. **Provision and coordination of care:** This domain relates to the coordination, organisation and provision of nursing care. It includes the assessment of individuals or groups, planning, implementation and evaluation of care within a clinical reasoning framework.

4. **Collaborative and therapeutic practice:** This domain refers to establishing, sustaining and concluding professional and therapeutic relationships with individuals or groups. This domain also contains those competencies that relate to a nurse's ability to communicate and collaborate with members of the interprofessional healthcare team.

See the section on reflective practice in Chapter 4 for an example of how these competency standards inform nursing students' clinical practice.

Code of ethics for Australian nurses

The *Code of ethics for nurses in Australia* (NMBA 2008a) outlines the nursing profession's commitment to respect, promote, protect and uphold the fundamental rights of people who are both the recipients and providers of nursing and healthcare. It complements the International Council of Nurses *Code of ethics for nurses* (2012) and the New Zealand Nurses Organisation *Code of ethics* (2010).

The purpose of the *Code of ethics* for nurses in Australia is to:

- identify the fundamental ethical standards and values to which the nursing profession is committed and that are incorporated in other endorsed professional nursing guidelines and standards of conduct
- provide nurses with a reference point from which to reflect on themselves and on others
- guide ethical decision making and practice
- indicate to the community the human rights standards and ethical values it can expect nurses to uphold.

Value statements that comprise the code of ethics include:

- Nurses value quality nursing care for all people.
- Nurses value respect and kindness for themselves and others.
- Nurses value the diversity of people.
- Nurses value access to quality nursing and healthcare for all people.
- Nurses value informed decision making.
- Nurses value a culture of safety in nursing and healthcare.
- Nurses value ethical management of information.
- Nurses value a socially, economically and ecologically sustainable environment that promotes health and wellbeing.

See the section 'Ethical dilemmas in nursing' in Chapter 4 for an example of how these ethical standards inform nurses' clinical practice.

Code of conduct for Australian nurses

The *Code of professional conduct for nurses in Australia* (NMBA 2008b) sets the minimum standards for practice a professional nurse is expected to uphold, both within and outside of professional domains, in order to ensure the 'good standing' of the nursing profession. The code of conduct provides a framework for legally and professionally accountable nursing practice in all clinical, managerial, educational and research-based domains.

According to the code of conduct a nurse must:

- practise in a safe and competent manner
- practise in accordance with the agreed standards of the profession and broader health system
- practise and conduct themselves in accordance with laws relevant to the profession and practice of nursing
- respect the dignity, culture, ethnicity, values and beliefs of people receiving care and treatment, and that of other colleagues
- treat personal information obtained in a professional capacity as private and confidential
- provide impartial, honest and accurate information in relation to nursing care and healthcare products
- support the health, wellbeing and informed decision making of people who require or are receiving care
- promote and preserve the trust and privilege inherent in the relationship between nurses and people who receive care
- maintain and build upon the community's trust and confidence in the nursing profession
- practise nursing reflectively and ethically.

If you practise in Australia then it is essential that you become very familiar with the NMBA codes, guidelines and statements. We provide only the briefest overview of these standards here. The full documents are available from the NMBA website at <www.nursingmidwiferyboard.gov.au>.

Similarly, if you are a nursing student in New Zealand, we encourage you to become familiar with the standards and guidelines for nurses available from the Nursing Council of New Zealand at <www.nursingcouncil.org.nz> and from the New Zealand Nurses Organisation at <www.nzno.org.nz>.

LEGAL REQUIREMENTS

In addition to professional expectations, nurses and nursing students must understand and comply with the legal principles that govern their practice. You will cover these in detail in your nursing program. In the next section we provide brief explanations of privacy and confidentiality, two legal principles that nursing students often find difficult to understand and apply to their practice.

Privacy and confidentiality
Privacy

Government legislation requires that health professionals protect the personal information and privacy of others. This legislation ensures that information about people is not used without their consent. Privacy is a right for all individuals, and you need to ensure you understand your obligations in respect of privacy laws.

Disclosure of personal health information: This refers to communicating or transferring information outside a health service, giving a copy of or excerpt from personal health information to another organisation or individual, allowing another organisation or individual to have access to the information, or communicating the information in any other way.

Health or medical record: This is a documented account, whether in hard or electronic form, of a client's health, illness and treatment during a visit or stay at a health service.

Personal health information: Any personal information collected for the purposes of providing healthcare will generally be classified as 'personal health information'. It includes information or an opinion about a person's:

- physical or mental health or illness
- wishes about the future provision of health services
- receipt or record of health services.

Personal information: This includes unique identifying information such as a client's name, address, date of birth, ethnicity, diagnosis, photographs and biometric information (including fingerprints and genetic characteristics).

Patients should be informed that their personal health information will be protected and that it will be given to another person only if it is essential to their healthcare or can be otherwise legally and ethically justified. You are obliged to protect and maintain personal information about your patients during clinical placements. Personal information is any information that can identify a person. Health information (e.g. health records) is also protected. Information about individuals must not be given to others without the individual's consent. This includes the giving of personal information to relatives and friends during phone calls or in face-to-face conversations.

SOMETHING TO THINK ABOUT

A man was admitted for a vasectomy unbeknown to his partner who was a ward clerk in another part of the hospital. A 'well-meaning' nurse informed the man's partner when he returned from surgery, to let her know his condition. Needless to say the situation did not end well for any of the people involved.

Nursing students are usually required to sign a privacy or confidentiality undertaking and must comply with privacy law and policies. Students are usually given access to health records with the approval of their clinical supervisor if the information is directly relevant to their learning. Access does not include photocopying or transcribing records that contain personal health information, or taking such records offsite. Clients/patients have the right to refuse permission for students to access their records and many facilities require patients to sign a written consent form before students can use patient information for something like a case study.

The anonymity of clients/patients should be maintained during debriefing, case studies and/or presentations, seminars and conferences. Use of photos, slides and other visual aids that identify individuals should not occur. Any information used should be with the client's permission and be de-identified.

Coaching tips

- Be aware of what constitutes privacy and what is considered to be a breach of privacy.
- Protect your patient's privacy throughout all nursing care activities.
- Remember that access to any patient information, including patient notes, requires permission.
- Only collect the minimum amount of information about a person after obtaining their consent.
- Seek advice and guidance about policies and protocols in operation at each facility where you undertake a placement. These will vary depending on the type of facility and its policies, guidelines and directives.
- Refrain from writing blogs and using social media to discuss your patients, staff, fellow students or other aspects of your placement. These activities can lead to breach of a person's privacy and have legal consequences (see 'Use of social media' in Chapter 5 for more information about the use of social media).

SOMETHING TO THINK ABOUT

Responsibility for sensitive confidential information about clients or patients is both a burden and a privilege for carers, but it also gives them a special relationship with those in their care and a subtle power over them.

Source: Thompson et al. 2006, p. 119

Confidentiality

Confidentiality is a broad concept that extends the concept of privacy. Although nurses may discuss personal details and care related to patients, this discussion should be constrained by ethical standards and responsible judgement. Nursing codes specify that nurses must treat as confidential personal information obtained in a professional capacity (NMBA 2008b; Nursing Council of New Zealand 2012a).

People often disclose sensitive and private information about themselves to health professionals. However, in doing so, patients make themselves vulnerable. Patient vulnerability is protected by the legal principles and practices of confidentiality. When information is required for educational, quality improvement or research purposes, informed consent must be provided and the anonymity of patients protected.

Confidentiality can be defined as a professional obligation to respect privileged information between health provider and client. Consider the following story.

STUDENT STORY
'Shhh ... keep your voice down'
Nathan's story

Nathan was in the hospital coffee shop when his fellow nursing students wandered over to join him. They were excited about having witnessed the birth of a baby and wanted to share their experiences. However, Nathan felt uncomfortable when one of his peers began to speak explicitly about processes related to the delivery, complications that had occurred, and the name of the new baby. Nathan cautioned his colleagues about maintaining confidentiality and said, 'Shhh ... keep your voice down', so that people nearby could not hear. While his colleagues were initially annoyed about being criticised and felt somewhat belittled by Nathan's comments, they soon realised his intent and complied.

Coaching tips

- Do not use patient experiences as 'conversation pieces'. Disclosing even snippets of information may breach confidentiality and assist a listener to identify a person.
- Confidentiality means that you need to consider how information is used, handled, stored or restricted. Always dispose of patient lists and handover notes taken during your shift in line with the institution's policies and in a way that ensures no information that can identify the client is visible or accessible.

SPEAK UP, SPEAK OUT

So far we have discussed patients' and clinicians' expectations of nursing students and professional and legal requirements. Now we move to personal expectations. Students often have unrealistic and unattainable expectations of their performance when on clinical placement and are sometimes their own worse critics. Compounding these expectations is the cognitive dissonance that can arise when students' expectations, beliefs or principles are compromised and they feel powerless to speak out.

Standing up for what you believe is one of the most important aspects of personal integrity. Yet speaking up or speaking out in clinical contexts is not always easy. Decades ago, nursing students were socialised to obedience, respect for authority and loyalty to the team. Their acceptance into, and continued membership of, the healthcare team depended upon their recognition of this subordinate role (Kelly 1996). Nearly a century ago Florence Nightingale described the qualities of a 'good nurse' as 'restraint, discipline and obedience', adding that the nurse should 'carry out the orders of the doctors in a suitably humble and deferential way ... and obey to the letter the requirements of the matron and the sister' (Baly 1991, p. 11). Society expected nurses to be submissive, subordinate, humble and self-sacrificing. Within the hierarchy of the healthcare system, nurses became acculturated to do and say what was expected, to conform rather than to question, to accept rather than debate important issues (Levett-Jones & Lathlean 2009).

This outdated image no longer defines nursing. However, even though nurses are expected to speak out against poor practice or to challenge ethical or legal issues, some students find this difficult, especially when they believe their acceptance into the team may hinge on their conformity to it. Wanting to fit in and be accepted is a fundamental and universal motivation (Levett-Jones 2007); however, when fitting in becomes more important than doing what is right, it can become an ethical dilemma. The greatest threat to personal integrity is silence in the face of perceived wrong. We sometimes fail to consider the price of silence. To know something is wrong and to say nothing indirectly consents to what has occurred. In doing nothing we become part of the problem. This presents an enormous dilemma for students. By speaking out you may risk ridicule, rejection or social isolation. By not speaking out you may compromise your integrity and patient safety.

STUDENT STORY
'I have seen things and not said anything'
Nicole's story

Nicole, a mature-age student, described how she became increasingly confident of her place in the nursing environment as she progressed through her program, and because of that became more willing to challenge poor practice:

I have seen things and not said anything. That has changed as my confidence and knowledge have grown. I still remember seeing two healthcare assistants pulling an elderly woman up the bed in the most hideous manner and not saying anything to them, but now I would definitely say something.

Source: Levett-Jones & Lathlean 2009

SOMETHING TO THINK ABOUT
To everything there is a season, and a time to every purpose under heaven: a time to keep silence, and a time to speak.
Ecclesiastes 3:1

Many situations present ethical dilemmas for student nurses. Horizontal violence (or bullying), unsafe clinical practice or breaches of legal and/or ethical standards may require you to take a stand and to speak out. How will you respond? What will you say?

The ability to state your opinion clearly and honestly without offending anyone requires great skill. Start by using 'I' statements. Griffin (2004) provides some excellent examples of 'I' statements:

- 'I don't feel right talking about him/her when I wasn't there and I don't know all the facts.'
- 'I'm not prepared to talk about it because it was shared in confidence.'
- 'I don't think that was what really happened—let's ask the people involved.'

Concerns about patient-care standards are just as challenging and often need to be interpreted in consultation with an experienced and objective support person, such as your clinical educator. Be cautious though; sometimes what may seem at first to be poor practice may not be so when interpreted in the light of all the facts. Don't react without some guidance and knowledge of all pertinent issues. You can still use 'I' statements, but be tactful in your approach. 'I don't understand the reason for that decision' is often a wise opening statement that allows for lines of communication to remain open and for explanations to be provided. (Refer to Chapter 3 for information about advocating for and on behalf of patients.)

There may come a time when you feel you must speak out strongly against a clinical, ethical or professional issue. Make sure you are guided by the relevant *code of ethics* (NMBA 2008a; New Zealand Nurses Organisation 2010). As a student you may need to call upon your support networks, clinical educators or university staff for guidance and advice. In some situations they may need to advocate on your behalf.

Speaking up or speaking out is an act of moral courage. It often comes at cost. But an even greater cost comes with silence—the loss of self-respect. The benefits of speaking up outweigh the risks, not only from a personal point of view but also from a professional perspective (Hedley 2007). When in doubt about whether you should speak out, reflect on the words of Martin Luther King Jr: 'He who passively accepts evil is as much involved in it as he who helps to perpetrate it. He who accepts evil without protesting against it is really cooperating with it' (Corporation for National and Community Service 2014).

DON'T TAKE THINGS PERSONALLY

The clinical learning environment is a complex social setting and can present many challenges to students. Some of these you will find exhilarating, and others will provide you with experiences that will improve your interpersonal skills. Accepting constructive feedback from staff and educators about your behaviour during challenging situations will add to your growth and development. When things go wrong or you've made a mistake and the feedback you receive is difficult to hear, avoid taking things personally. Consider each situation as a clinical issue or problem, rather than something that is a personal attack or problem for you. Remember that all situations create learning opportunities, and through learning we change and grow, develop new skill sets, knowledge and attitudes, and re-evaluate our belief systems.

Consider the example below of a student who demonstrated less than appropriate professional behaviour following a directive from her clinical educator.

STUDENT STORY
'It's not fair …'
Evelyn's story

Evelyn wanted to spend time in the operating theatre, but she was told by her clinical educator that she was to remain on the medical ward because the perioperative unit already had a group of students. During her lunch break, Evelyn found out that another student in her group had been to theatre that morning with her patient. She went to her clinical educator and complained that she had stopped her from achieving one of her goals and that she was favouring other students. Discussions about the situation between Evelyn and her clinical educator became strained when Evelyn could not understand why she couldn't go to the unit when her colleague had done so. Evelyn saw the issue as one of unfairness and took it personally. She then complained to university staff about the way she was treated by the clinical educator.

On examination of the issues surrounding the complaint, the university staff identified that eight students from another university were allocated to the perioperative environment. Students from the ward locations were permitted to visit the perioperative environment only if they accompanied the surgical patients they were caring for. As Evelyn was on a medical ward, none of her patients were scheduled for the operating theatre.

The very nature of the clinical environment is dynamic and so each student's learning experience will be different. It is not beneficial to compare your experiences and opportunities to those of other students, as no two experiences will ever be the same. In the above situation, Evelyn's placement did not give her the opportunity to go to the perioperative unit and the decision taken by the educator was a professional one, not a personal one.

- Identify challenging or difficult situations and work through them using conflict-resolution strategies (see Chapter 3).
- Be aware of your own behaviours, how you react to situations and how you work through issues.
- Seek assistance from mentors, educators and other relevant staff, as necessary, to work through situations in the clinical learning environment.

COMPLIANCE AND COMPROMISE

In this section we consider the importance of belonging but delve into the 'dark side' of this phenomenon for nursing students. A broad range of psychological literature describes the importance of belonging, as well as the negative emotional, psychological, physical and behavioural consequences of having this need thwarted (Levett-Jones & Lathlean 2009). The absence of meaningful interpersonal work relationships can lead to unquestioning agreement with other people's decisions, acquiescence, compliance or going along with negative behaviours sanctioned by group members, often in order to belong (Sedgwick 2013).

What does this mean for you? For some students, the need to belong and to be accepted into the team is more important than the quality of care they provide and the level of competency they aspire to (Levett-Jones & Lathlean 2009). Reread that sentence and ask yourself if it could apply to you. Nursing students have described how they sometimes go along with clinical practices that they know to be wrong so as not to 'rock the boat'. They share how it is easier to just accept that 'this is the way it is done here' rather than be labelled a 'troublemaker' (Levett-Jones & Lathlean 2009). Compare these notions with what you've learnt about questioning practices that are not evidence-based.

STUDENT STORY
Conformity and compromise: personal and professional implications
Lei's story

This story demonstrates how an international student complied with the directives of her mentor in order to be accepted by the nursing staff she worked with, even though doing so put her patient at risk.

One registered nurse that I was buddied up with asked me to shower a patient who was blind and I said, 'Okay, no problem', and went in and started the shower. Then the nurse asked me to do something else while the patient was in the shower. I said, 'I can't really leave her here by herself, she's blind. Can I at least finish and make sure she's safe?' But the nurse said, 'She showers herself at home, you don't need to be there. I need

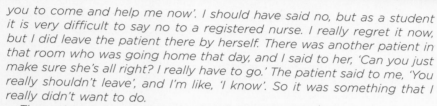

STUDENT STORY *cont'd*

you to come and help me now'. I should have said no, but as a student it is very difficult to say no to a registered nurse. I really regret it now, but I did leave the patient there by herself. There was another patient in that room who was going home that day, and I said to her, 'Can you just make sure she's all right? I really have to go.' The patient said to me, 'You really shouldn't leave', and I'm like, 'I know'. So it was something that I really didn't want to do.

The patient got up, tried to get out of the shower on her own and water went everywhere. The nurse unit manager found her like that, blind, naked and shivering, with water everywhere. She said, 'Who left you here?' She found out it was me and said, 'What do you think you are doing? You should know better than this. You're in second year, you should know this.' I just said, 'I'm really sorry, I should have known.' I wanted to take responsibility because the nurse unit manager was telling me that in front of all the patients. So I said, 'I'm really sorry, it won't happen again. I should have known better'—and then I was furious inside; I was upset. I tried to forget about it; these things happen. But this memory has really stuck in my mind.

Source: Levett-Jones 2007

Coaching tips

We would like to give you a tried-and-tested recipe for overcoming the need to conform in order to belong, but really there is no simple solution. We advise you to reflect on this section thoughtfully. At some stage you may be in a situation where you'll feel pressured to compromise your practice. Think carefully about the consequences—for you and for your patient.

EXERCISE YOUR RIGHTS

On campus and in clinical placements, you'll hear a great deal about expectations and responsibilities. Always keep in mind that alongside responsibilities there are also rights. Nurses have focused on their responsibilities for so long that they are often surprised at the prospect of having rights themselves. Rights always seem to belong to other people—human rights, patients' rights, women's rights, consumer rights—the list goes on. It's time to think about your rights as a nursing student. In the *Coaching tips* below we touch on a few of your rights and provide some strategies to help you to exercise these rights.

1. The right to ask questions

As a student your primary purpose in undertaking a clinical placement is to learn. This won't happen unless you ask questions. Most of the nurses you work with will welcome your questions and the opportunity to support your learning. Unfortunately, you will sometimes encounter nurses who are less receptive to your questions.

It's your right to ask questions, but always ask at the right time and in the right place. To develop your critical thinking and clinical reasoning skills, attempt to work through the question first and develop a tentative answer. For example, if you're concerned about your patient's fluid status you could say to your mentor, 'I've assessed Mrs Smith's fluid status—her urine output has been less than 20 mL per hour for the past three hours, her specific gravity is high, blood pressure 100/60, pulse 110, weak and thready, her mucous membranes are dry and her tongue furrowed. I think she is dehydrated. She has an intravenous infusion currently running TKVO. Should we contact the medical officer for a review of her fluid orders?' Taking this approach allows you to think through the problem, practise clinical reasoning, demonstrate initiative and ask informed questions.

2. The right to question practice

This is a right that nursing students don't always exercise. You will learn about 'best practice' and 'evidence-based healthcare' (and we discuss it in Chapter 3), but at times you will see nursing practice that seems to be based on little more than authority ('the doctor said to do it this way'), tradition ('we've always done it this way') and local policy ('this is the way we do it here'). You may find yourself placed in a confusing and somewhat uncomfortable position with this contradiction between evidence and practice.

3. The right to refuse (without feeling guilty or making excuses)

Often when students refuse a request from a superior they feel guilty and uncomfortable, even when they are within their rights, and even when it is their responsibility to refuse. Here is an example in which a student refused, politely and tactfully, but with determination:

Registered nurse: 'Can you please administer the oral medications to the patient in room 11? You're in third year so I trust you to do this.'

Student: 'Thank you for trusting me to do this on my own, but as a student I'm required to have the administration of all medications counter-checked and countersigned by the nurse responsible for the patient's care. What you're asking me to do is outside of my scope of practice and I can fail my clinical placement if I do what you've asked.'

Remember also that 'the right to refuse' is the sixth medication right!

Coaching tips (cont'd)

4. The right to be supernumerary to the workforce

Since nursing education moved to universities students have undertaken clinical placements in a supernumerary capacity. This means that you are not part of the workforce but are there in addition to the employed staff. This is so your learning is not compromised by the demands and responsibilities of patient care. However, occasionally students, particularly when in their third year, are used to fill a gap in the roster. While we encourage students to take a patient load, it should always be in a supernumerary capacity and under the supervision of the nurse responsible for the patient's care. If this situation presents itself, politely explain your university's policy and, if the situation is not resolved, contact your facilitator or university support person.

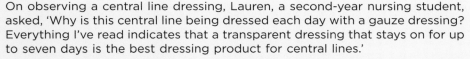

STUDENT STORY

Why is it being dressed that way?
Lauren's story

On observing a central line dressing, Lauren, a second-year nursing student, asked, 'Why is this central line being dressed each day with a gauze dressing? Everything I've read indicates that a transparent dressing that stays on for up to seven days is the best dressing product for central lines.'

Lauren's comment promoted a lot of dialogue and debate among the registered nurses and doctors. Not too much later, following a review of the literature, the central-line dressing regimen was updated at that hospital and transparent dressings are now used.

Remember: When questioning practice, be tactful and polite; there may be very sound reasons for the way nursing procedures are undertaken.

References

Australian Commission on Safety and Quality in Health Care. *A guide for consumers, carers and families.* Online. Available: <http://www.hqcc.qld.gov.au/Resources/Documents/Brochure-Australian-Charter-of-Healthcare-Rights-A-guide-for-consumers-carers-and-families-English-Jan-2012.pdf>; 2012 Accessed 15.01.14.

Baly M. *As Miss Nightingale said ...* London: Scutari Press; 1991.

Corporation for National and Community Service. *Rev. Dr Martin Luther King, Jr. quotes.* Online. Available: <http://mlkday.gov/plan/library/communications/quotes.php>; 2014 Accessed 27.05.14.

Griffin M. Teaching cognitive rehearsal as a shield for lateral violence: an intervention for newly licensed nurses. *J Contin Educ Nurs.* 2004;35(6):257-264.

Hedley T. *Sick to death.* Crows Nest: Allen & Unwin; 2007.

International Council of Nurses. *Code of ethics for nurses.* Online. Available: <www.icn.ch/about-icn/code-of-ethics-for-nurses>; 2012 Accessed 15.01.14.

Kelly B. Speaking up: a moral obligation. *Nurs Forum.* 1996;31(2):31-34.

Levett-Jones T. *Belongingness: a pivotal precursor to optimising the learning of nursing students in the clinical environment.* Unpublished PhD thesis. Newcastle: The University of Newcastle; 2007.

Levett-Jones T, Lathlean J. 'Don't rock the boat': nursing students' experiences of conformity and compliance. *Nurse Educ Today*. 2009;29(3):342-349.

McCormack B, McCance T, Slater P, et al. Person-centred outcomes and cultural change. In: Manley K, McCormack B, Wilson V, eds. *International practice development in nursing and healthcare*. Oxford: Blackwell Publishing; 2008:189-214.

McIlfatrick S, Sullivan K, McKenna H, et al. Patient's experiences of having chemotherapy in a day hospital setting. *J Adv Nurs*. 2007;59(3):264-273. <http://www.ncbi.nlm.nih.gov/pubmed?term=Parahoo%20K%5B Author%5D&cauthor=true&cauthor_uid=17590208>.

New South Wales Health, Nursing and Midwifery Office. *Essentials of Care project*. Online. Available: <http://www.health.nsw.gov.au/nursing/projects/Pages/eoc.aspx>; 2009 Accessed 15.01.14.

New Zealand Nurses Organisation. *Code of ethics*. Online. Available: <www.nzno.org.nz/resources/nzno_publications>; 2010 Accessed 09.01.14.

Nursing and Midwifery Board of Australia (NMBA). *National competency standards for the registered nurse*. Online. Available: <www.nursingmidwiferyboard.gov.au>; 2006 Accessed 15.01.14.

Nursing and Midwifery Board of Australia (NMBA). *National competency standards for the enrolled nurse*. Online. Available: <www.nursingmidwiferyboard.gov.au>; 2002 Accessed 14.04.14.

Nursing and Midwifery Board of Australia (NMBA). *Code of ethics for nurses in Australia*. Online. Available: <www.nursingmidwiferyboard.gov.au>; 2008a Accessed 15.01.14.

Nursing and Midwifery Board of Australia (NMBA). *Code of professional conduct for nurses in Australia*. Online. Available: <www.nursingmidwiferyboard.gov.au>; 2008b Accessed 15.01.14.

Nursing Council of New Zealand. *Competencies for registered nurses*. Online. Available: <http://nursingcouncil.org.nz/Publications/Standards-and-guidelines-for-nurses>; 2007 Accessed 09.01.14.

Nursing Council of New Zealand. *Code of conduct for nurses*. Online. Available: <www.nursingcouncil.org.nz/Nurses/Code-of-Conduct>; 2012a Accessed 09.01.14.

Nursing Council of New Zealand. *Guidelines for cultural safety, the Treaty of Waitangi and Maori health*. Online. Available: <www.nursingcouncil.org.nz/Publications/Standards-and-guidelines-for-nurses>; 2011b Accessed 15.01.14.

Sedgwick M. Comparison of second-degree and traditional undergraduate nursing students' sense of belonging during clinical placements. *J Nurs Educ*. 2013;52:657-661.

Thompson IE, Melia KM, Boyd KM, et al. *Nursing ethics*. Edinburgh: Churchill Livingstone; 2006.

How you act

Actions speak louder than words

Proverb

INTRODUCTION

In this chapter we focus on students' actions and behaviour when undertaking clinical placements. We avoid being too prescriptive but instead profile authentic clinical scenarios to help you consider the potential consequences of your actions. We also explore some of the more difficult situations that students may have to deal with, such as sexual harassment, bullying and conflict with peers. Our aim is to fortify you so that if you encounter any of these negative and distressing situations you will have an armoury of strategies to help deal with them. Our thinking is that 'forewarned is forearmed'.

CULTURAL COMPETENCE

SOMETHING TO THINK ABOUT

I went to have some blood tests. The person doing the test was asking me questions but I couldn't understand anything. There was no interpreter. I couldn't ask for one because I don't speak any English. Some days later they called me on the mobile. He was talking in English. I tried to get someone off the street to listen and translate but the doctor just kept talking, talking and then hung up the phone. I don't know how to get the results of my tests.

Source: Brough 2006, p. 14

Culture refers to a shared set of values, ideas, concepts and rules of group behaviour. Culture includes, but is not limited to: age or generation; gender; sexual orientation; occupation and socioeconomic status; ethnic origin or migrant experience; and religious or spiritual beliefs. The aspects of culture we can easily see in others (e.g. food, dress and language) are like the tip of an iceberg; the majority is hidden from view, and largely unknown (Gilligan et al. 2014).

With a population originating from 160 countries, where 200 languages are spoken and 116 religions practised (Seaton 2010), Australia is among the most culturally diverse nations in the world (National Health and Medical Research Council 2005). Immigration has contributed almost half of the population growth in Australia in recent years, with one in four Australian residents born overseas (Australian Bureau of Statistics 2012). This increase in cultural diversity has placed greater emphasis on nurses' ability and willingness to provide culturally competent care.

Culturally and linguistically diverse (CALD) patients are twice as likely to experience serious adverse outcomes as English-speaking people (Multicultural Health Communication 2013). Reports describe misunderstandings, miscommunication and cultural assumptions in the care of CALD patients. A body of research indicates that CALD people experience poorer pain assessment and treatment and a higher incidence of misdiagnosis and wrong surgery due to language barriers (Johnstone & Kanitsaki 2006). CALD people access health services less often, and when they do fewer diagnostic procedures are performed (Multicultural Health Communication 2013). CALD people also report feelings of powerlessness, loneliness and fear when undergoing healthcare (Garrett et al. 2008). While there is no single cause of the inequities in health and healthcare experienced by CALD groups, studies have linked adverse patient outcomes to clinical encounters that do not acknowledge and address cultural factors (Johnstone & Kanitsaki 2008).

'Cultural competence is a set of congruent behaviours, attitudes and policies that come together in a system, agency or among professionals and enable that system, agency or those professionals to work effectively in cross-cultural situations' (Cross et al. 1989). Cultural competence is much more than awareness of cultural differences, as it focuses on the capacity of the health system to improve health and wellbeing by integrating culture into the delivery of health services (Eisenbruch 2004). Culturally competent nurses are able to deliver safe care to all people regardless of their race, ethnicity, culture or language proficiency (Kramer et al. 1998). A nurse who is culturally competent (see Box 3.1) engages in assistive, supportive, facilitative or enabling acts that are tailored to fit with individual, group or cultural values, beliefs and worldviews, to provide safe and quality healthcare (Lehman et al. n.d.).

Cultural competence is linked to improved patient care (Paez et al. 2009) and reduced adverse outcomes (Fernadez et al. 2012). Culturally competent healthcare leads to increases in health-seeking behaviour, more appropriate screening and testing, fewer clinical reasoning errors, greater adherence to medical advice, reduced medication errors, and the provision of person-centred care (Lehman et al. n.d.).

The Nursing and Midwifery Board of Australia (NMBA) *National competency standards for the registered nurse* (NMBA 2006) specify that competent nurses recognise that ethnicity, culture, gender, spiritual values, sexuality, age, disability and economic and social factors have an impact on an individual's responses to, and beliefs about, health and illness. The competency standards also state that nurses should plan and modify nursing care appropriately, and accept individuals/groups regardless of race, culture, religion, age, gender, sexual preference, physical or mental state.

Nurses who are culturally competent engage in the following behaviours:

- facilitating effective communication by using interpreters or bilingual health staff
- negotiating the nature and extent of family involvement
- seeking to understand a patient's beliefs, expectations and experiences
- being compassionate and respecting patient and human rights (by holding regular, open conversations directly with patients and their families in order to demonstrate empathy, kindness and respect)
- negotiating a care partnership by exploring the patient's and family's view of the cause of the illness, when how and why it started, its severity, the expected treatment and results
- providing services such as multilingual signage and a range of food options, and facilitating access to religious leaders (Garrett et al. 2008).

Box 3.1 Attributes of a culturally competent nurse

Awareness
- Knowledge of self and awareness of own culture
- Understanding that people have different frameworks, and that one can't possibly know everything about every culture

Attitudes
- Willingness to learn and curiosity about others
- Humility

Knowledge
- Of the organisation's policies, protocols, resources (e.g. knowing when and how to access interpreters or multicultural liaison officers)
- Of your patient and their history
- Of the social and political environment the patient has come from
- Of non-verbal cues (e.g. eye contact, smiling and silence can mean different things to different people)

Source: Gilligan et al. 2014

One of the most important ways of ensuring culturally competent care is by undertaking a cultural assessment. This includes asking questions such as:

- What do you think has caused your illness?
- Why do you think your illness started when it did?
- What kind of treatment do you think you should receive?
- What are the most important results you hope to receive from this treatment?
- What are the main problems your illness has caused you?
- What do you fear most about your illness?
- How can your family be helpful to you in dealing with your illness?
- Who is the decision-maker in your family regarding healthcare issues?
- How can we support your spiritual needs and practices?

SOMETHING TO THINK ABOUT

We often assume that everyone who looks or sounds the same *is* the same. However, individuals from culturally diverse populations have differing skills, knowledge and values. It is essential to understand people as individuals within the context of cultural competence.

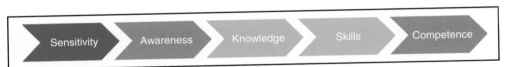

Figure 3.1 The process of gaining cultural competence

Cultural competence can be viewed as a process (see Figure 3.1), with clear differences between each stage (Table 3.1).

Table 3.1 Understanding the difference between cultural awareness, sensitivity, competence and safety

Cultural sensitivity	A process of recognising the attitudes, values, beliefs and practices within your own culture so you can have an insight into your effect on others
Cultural awareness	Knowledge, understanding and appreciating difference and diversity; recognising that we do not always have a shared history or a shared understanding of the present
Cultural competence	Providing effective and appropriate, positive and empowering care to all
Cultural safety	Supports a social justice approach to healthcare; cultural safety is specific to working in a cross-cultural context with Indigenous people

Ellis et al. (2010), Kikuchi (2005), ANMC and Nursing Council of New Zealand (2010), Schim et al. (2005).

Another frequently used term in Australia and New Zealand is 'cultural safety'. The Nursing Council of New Zealand defines cultural safety as the 'effective nursing practice of a person or family from another culture as determined by that person or family' (2011, p. 7). Cultural safety is a term that is often used when referring to the care of Indigenous peoples. Culturally safe care for Indigenous peoples requires nurses to possess:

- awareness of important Indigenous issues, such as cultural differences, specific aspects of Indigenous history and its impact on Indigenous peoples in contemporary society
- the skills to interact and communicate sensitively and effectively
- the desire or motivation to be successful in their interactions with Indigenous peoples, in order to improve access, service delivery and client outcomes (Farrelly & Lumby 2009).

SOMETHING TO THINK ABOUT

- When we treat people *equally* we ignore differences.
- When we treat people *equitably* we recognise and respect differences.

Coaching tips

- Reflect on and come to know and understand your own values and culture.
- Consider the assumptions, power imbalances, attitudes and beliefs you hold that are different from those of others.
- Learn about and engage in a social justice agenda.
- Seek to understand the cultural beliefs and practices of other people.
- Understand that effective communication is essential to culturally competent care, and work to develop these skills.
- Be attuned to non-verbal communication (body language), silence and touch.
- Tailor your care to meet patients' social, cultural, religious and linguistic needs as stated by the patient.
- Provide effective nursing care by working in partnership with your patients.
- Use trained interpreters for care requirements when language barriers are evident.
- Accept and value difference and diversity in human behaviour, social structure and culture.

SOMETHING TO THINK ABOUT

Mrs Tainui was a Maori woman who had been diagnosed with lung cancer. She had been admitted to hospital for palliative care. Within a few days the cancerous lesions had grown significantly. She began to experience difficulty in breathing and underwent a procedure to remove fluid from her lungs. She found the pleurocentesis (fluid tap procedure) very painful. Her doctor explained that the cancer was extremely fast growing, and she was offered radiotherapy and chemotherapy. She was advised that these approaches would give her a little more time but would not save her life.

Mrs Tainui considered the treatment options and their associated side effects and discussed the issues with her daughters. Her main concern was the loss of hair that would result from the chemotherapy. Her cultural traditions included the belief that she must die as a whole person. She believed that without her hair she could not be considered to be a whole person. Together with her family's blessing, Mrs Tainui declined the treatment that may have afforded her a longer life so she could die according to her cultural identity.

What are your thoughts about Mrs Tainui's decision? Consider how your practice would demonstrate cultural competence if you were the nurse caring for Mrs Tainui.

PATIENT SAFETY

Patient safety is considered to be one of the most important issues facing healthcare today. Healthcare is increasingly complex; this complexity, coupled with inherent human performance limitations, even in experienced, skilled and committed health professionals, means that some clinical errors are almost inevitable. However, when seeking healthcare, people hope and trust that their health-related problems will be appropriately managed and that their care will be safe and effective (Levett-Jones 2014). Yet, despite the best intentions of health professionals, a seminal study identified that between 10% and 16% of patients are harmed while receiving healthcare (Wilson et al. 1995), resulting in distress, hospital admissions, permanent injury, increased length of hospital stay, and death. Importantly, more than 50% of these adverse events are preventable (Weingart & Wilson 2000).

Patient safety is defined as actions undertaken by individuals and organisations to protect healthcare recipients from being harmed by their healthcare (National Patient Safety Foundation 2014). It is important to note that patient safety is not limited to physical safety but also includes psychological, emotional and cultural safety. Patient safety is an attribute of trustworthy healthcare systems that work to minimise the incidence and impact of, and maximise recovery from, adverse events (Emanuel et al. 2008).

Health professionals need a sound knowledge base and well-developed clinical skills in order to manage the complex health needs and competing tensions evident in contemporary practice environments (Levett-Jones et al. 2014). However, knowledge and skills alone will not result in improved patient outcomes. Nearly 60% of the adverse patient outcomes are caused by clinical reasoning errors (Wilson et al. 1995); this includes failure to collect, interpret and act on clinical data. Between 70% and 80% of errors are caused by ineffective communication between health professionals and the patients they care for, and among health professional themselves (Leonard et al. 2004). It is imperative therefore that nursing students take advantage of every opportunity to gain skills and knowledge while at the same time paying particular attention to ensuring they develop increasingly sophisticated clinical reasoning skills and the ability to communicate effectively.

The Australian Commission on Safety and Quality in Health Care has developed a set of safety and quality health service standards that focus on factors known to impact on patient safety. We list these standards in Box 3.2 so you gain a clear understanding of some of clinical issues that you need to become familiar with in order to make a difference to patient safety.

Box 3.2   National Safety and Quality Health Service Standards

Standard
Standard 1: Governance for safety and quality in health service organisations
Standard 2: Partnering with consumers
Standard 3: Preventing and controlling healthcare associated infection
Standard 4: Medication safety
Standard 5: Patient identification and procedure matching
Standard 6: Clinical handover
Standard 7: Blood and blood products
Standard 8: Preventing and managing pressure injuries
Standard 9: Recognising and responding to clinical deterioration in acute care
Standard 10: Preventing falls and harm from falls

Source: Australian Commission on Safety and Quality in Health Care 2014

All health professionals are committed to improving patient safety—indeed it is internationally recognised that 'patient safety is everybody's business'. For nurses this commitment is emphasised in the NMBA *National competency standards for the registered nurse* (NMBA 2006), which identifies that competent nurses:

- recognise and respond appropriately to unsafe or unprofessional practice
- participate in quality-improvement activities
- respond effectively to unexpected or rapidly changing situations
- facilitate a physical, psychosocial, cultural and spiritual environment that promotes individual and/or group safety and security.

Further, the NMBA *Code of ethics for nurses in Australia* (2008a) identifies in Value Statement 6 that nurses value a culture of safety in nursing and healthcare.

When thinking about the errors that happen in healthcare it is important not to adopt an overly simplistic approach. Rarely is an adverse event the result of one person or one error. There are multiple contextual and system-wide factors that create the conditions where errors can occur. It is helpful to consider Reason's 'Swiss cheese model' (Reason et al. 2001) when reviewing the causes of adverse events. In Reason's model of system failure every step in a process has the potential for failure, to varying degrees. The ideal system is like a stack of Swiss cheese slices. Each hole is an opportunity for a process to fail, and each slice is a 'defensive layer' in the process. An error may allow a problem to pass through a hole in one layer, but in the next layer the holes are in different places, and the problem should be caught. Each layer is a defence against the potential error. The fewer and smaller the holes, the more likely it is that an error will be caught or stopped. See Figure 3.2 for an example of how an adverse medication error can occur due to both human and system failures.

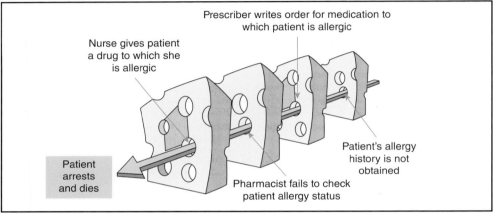

Prescriber writes order for medication to which patient is allergic

Nurse gives patient a drug to which she is allergic

Patient's allergy history is not obtained

Patient arrests and dies

Pharmacist fails to check patient allergy status

Figure 3.2 Reason's Swiss cheese model
Source: Reason, J. (2000)

Coaching tips

Learn all you can about patient safety and your role in preventing adverse patient events. Become familiar with the factors that impact on patient safety and how they can be prevented or managed. When you observe or are involved in a healthcare error carefully consider the factors that precipitated the error and how it could have been prevented

In Chapter 4 we introduce you to how critical thinking and clinical reasoning can have a positive impact on patient outcomes and in Chapter 5 we focus on communication as a way of improving patient safety. You can also access the following websites for further information about patient safety initiatives:

- Clinical Excellence Commission (www.cec.health.nsw.gov.au)

- Australian Commission on Safety and Quality in Health Care (www.safetyandquality.gov.au).

SOMETHING TO THINK ABOUT

In January 2004 Mr Graham Reeves was admitted to a hospital in the United Kingdom for removal of a badly diseased right kidney. A month before, he had seen the surgeon, who documented the need for removal of the right kidney in the patient's case notes. However, possibly due to a transcription error, the hospital admission slip wrongly said left kidney removal. This error was transcribed to the theatre list. One of the surgeons checked the x-ray in the operating theatre. But it was the wrong way around and he misread the diseased kidney as the one on the left. The second surgeon did not look at the x-ray. Early in the operation, a medical student looked at the x-ray and said she thought it was the right kidney that should be removed. The surgeon told her she had made a mistake and continued operating, removing the left kidney (the normal kidney). Mr Reeves died of kidney failure five weeks later. Had there been a greater culture of open communication where junior staff were encouraged to ask questions and where their concerns were taken seriously, Mr Reeves would not have died.

For other examples of how systems errors and a combination of inadequate technical and non-technical skills can lead to adverse patient outcomes, view the digital stories at <www.ipeforqum.com.au/modules>.

CLINICAL GOVERNANCE

Clinical governance is a systematic approach designed to improve and maintain safety and quality in healthcare (Sorensen & Iedema 2008; Wolff & Taylor 2009). It is an approach that encourages openness about strengths and weaknesses and incorporates the need to be proactive in order to improve clinical practice (Braithwaite & Travaglia 2008). Clinical governance requires accountability and responsibility for quality care and is about having the right people, policies, processes and information to be effective in delivering healthcare.

Many quality-improvement strategies are implemented in the clinical environment. You may be involved in initiatives such as clinical handover, chart audits and staff development activities, where clinical governance frameworks are used as a coordinating mechanism for improving quality care.

The guiding principles of clinical governance include:

- focusing on continuous quality improvement
- applying it to all facets of healthcare, across all service areas and models of practice, and including all healthcare providers
- developing partnerships between all people involved (patients and their families, managers, clinicians, students)
- learning from mistakes
- being open about failure
- emphasising learning
- developing a just culture in which individuals are treated fairly (Department of Health Government of Western Australia 2006; NSW Health 2005).

During clinical placements you will find evidence of clinical governance principles being implemented and will certainly be involved in different strategies. Each institution will interpret the principles differently and will implement strategies that have meaning and relevance to patients, the community and staff in that facility. For example, there will be: systems and infrastructures designed to ensure quality of care; guidelines or standards that govern practice; and mechanisms for data collection so that analysis and reports about care provision and services can be generated. In some cases these reports are linked directly to funding for the institution.

Some examples of clinical governance include:

- management of serious complaints
- performance reviews
- clinical audits
- management of incidents and accidents
- critical incident review
- clinical practice improvement programs (e.g. care pathways, standard setting)
- education, training and staff development programs
- accreditation and external quality reviews
- benchmarking processes
- policy generation.

BEST PRACTICE

SOMETHING TO THINK ABOUT

Often when we visit students on a clinical placement we ask them questions like 'What are you doing?', 'Why are you doing it?', 'Why are you doing it that way?' and 'Is there a better way?'. We're always thrilled if they can provide evidence-based justification for their practice. Too often nursing care is based upon little more than tradition or authority. As a nursing student you will learn how to practise nursing, some (hopefully most) of what you learn will be research-based. However, in 1997 Millenson estimated that 85% of healthcare practices were not scientifically validated. Over the past 10–20 years the nursing profession has given increased attention to evidence-based healthcare and a collage of information sources are now used to inform practice, each varying in dependability and validity.

The NMBA competency standards are very clear about the use of evidence to inform practice, stating that nurses should:

- identify the relevance of research to improving health outcomes
- identify problems in nursing practice that may be investigated through research
- discuss implications of research with colleagues
- participate in research

- use best available evidence, relevant literature and research findings to improve current practice
- demonstrate analytical skills in accessing and evaluating health information and research evidence
- undertake critical analysis of research findings.

Sources of evidence and knowledge
Tradition
In the nursing profession certain beliefs have been accepted as facts and certain practices accepted as effective, based purely on custom and tradition ('the way we've always done it'). These traditions and customs may be so entrenched that their use and usefulness is not questioned or rigorously evaluated. It is worrying when 'unit culture' ('the way it is done here') determines the way practice is undertaken, rather than basing clinical judgements on the best available evidence.

Authority
Another common source of knowledge is an authority figure—a person with specialised expertise or in a position of authority. Reliance on the advice of authority figures, such as nursing managers, educators or academics, is understandable. However, like tradition, these authorities as a source of information have limitations. Authorities are not infallible (especially if their knowledge is based mainly on personal experience), yet their views often go unchallenged.

Clinical experience
Clinical experience is a familiar and important source of knowledge. The ability to recognise regularities and irregularities, to generalise and to make predictions based on observations is a hallmark of good nursing practice. Nevertheless, this too has limitations; individual experiences and perspectives are sometimes narrow and biased.

Intuition
Nurses sometimes rely on 'intuition' in their practice. Intuition is a form of knowledge that cannot be explained on the basis of reasoning or prior instruction. Although intuition and 'hunches' can play a role in nursing practice, it is inappropriate to depend on these feelings alone as a source of evidence for practice. More reliable, however, is pattern-matching; this occurs when nurses use a collection of previous experiences to inform their current practice.

Trial and error
Sometimes nurses tackle problems by successively trying out alternative solutions. While this approach may be practical in some cases, it is often fallible and inefficient, to say nothing of the ethical implications of trial and error in clinical practice. This method tends to be haphazard, and the solutions are often idiosyncratic.

Assembled information
In making clinical decisions, healthcare professionals may use information that has been assembled for various purposes. For example, local, national and international benchmarking data provide information on the rates of various procedures and/or related complications (such as hospital-acquired infections). Risk-management data, such as critical incident reports and medication error reports, can be used to assess and measure improvements in practice. However, they do not always provide the actual information needed to implement practice improvement.

Evidence-based research

Nurses are increasingly expected to adopt an evidence-based practice approach, which can be defined as the use of the best clinical evidence available to inform patient care decisions. Evidence from rigorous studies constitutes the best type of evidence to underpin nurses' decisions and actions. Nursing care that is based on high-quality research evidence is more likely to be cost-effective and result in positive patient outcomes (Joanna Briggs Institute 2013).

The need for evidence to support practice has never been greater. The knowledge on which nursing care is based is constantly changing, and some of what you are taught in your nursing program will rapidly become obsolete. The volume of literature available to nurses is too large to stay continually up to date; transferring this research evidence into practice is sometimes difficult. For a nursing student, finding the best evidence for practice may seem daunting.

Fortunately, a lot of research has already been conducted, systematically reviewed and critically appraised. Websites such as that of the Joanna Briggs Institute and Cochrane Collaboration, among others, provide evidence for practice in easy-to-understand formats, such as systematic reviews and best-practice information sheets. These documents provide a summary of the best available evidence. Ask your librarian for advice about the best websites for accessing this type of quality research information.

SOMETHING TO THINK ABOUT

Every time you undertake nursing care or make a clinical decision, your action is based on something. Consider whether your actions are based on tradition, authority, trial and error, or intuition. It is your professional responsibility to ask, 'How do I know that this is really the most accurate decision or action?'.

ADVOCACY

Patient advocacy is an essential responsibility for all health professionals—it is no less an obligation for students. To be an advocate means that you empower and uphold the rights and interests of others. Patient advocacy is broadly defined as defending the rights of the vulnerable patient, or promoting the rights of others. The demonstration of competent practice requires nurses to 'advocate for individuals/groups when their rights are overlooked and/or compromised' (NMBA 2006). Ways to advocate for and to empower others include:

- informing a patient of her or his rights
- helping a patient to explore options
- helping a patient to help themselves
- speaking on behalf of a patient (if and when requested)
- assisting a patient to express their views clearly and confidently
- investigating and following up on complaints.

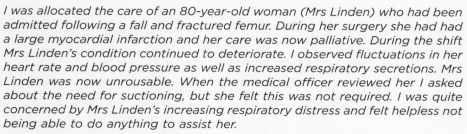

STUDENT STORY
The courage to advocate for a patient
Amy's story

I was allocated the care of an 80-year-old woman (Mrs Linden) who had been admitted following a fall and fractured femur. During her surgery she had had a large myocardial infarction and her care was now palliative. During the shift Mrs Linden's condition continued to deteriorate. I observed fluctuations in her heart rate and blood pressure as well as increased respiratory secretions. Mrs Linden was now unrousable. When the medical officer reviewed her I asked about the need for suctioning, but she felt this was not required. I was quite concerned by Mrs Linden's increasing respiratory distress and felt helpless not being able to do anything to assist her.

Mrs Linden's Cheyne-Stokes breathing continued and the secretions worsened. I sensed her time was near. I found this experience the most difficult in my student nursing career. I talked to her, applied lip balm, moisturised her skin and brushed her hair. I also noticed that she was beginning to grimace and groan.

I was unable to locate her blood pressure and heart rate. The medical officer retuned and ordered two more fluid boluses of 250 mL each. I was perplexed by this and respectfully asked why this was necessary because I thought comfort care was our goal. I felt this was futile and causing further distress to Mrs Linden. The medical officer changed the order to one bolus.

Not long after, Mrs Linden opened one eye and groaned. A tear rolled down her cheek. At this point I found the medical officer and, mindful of the doctrine of double effect, I told him what I had witnessed. He responded by saying, 'If you are telling me that the patient is in pain I will order her morphine'. 'Yes,' I replied, 'I feel she is in pain as evidenced by her groaning, grimacing and crying'.

Unfortunately the fluid bolus was still administered, but Mrs Linden also received morphine. Not long after, she passed away. The medical officer noticed my sadness and said, 'If that was my nan I would want you looking after her'. As I left that shift I was deeply saddened by the fact that Mrs Linden died without family or friends with her, but I felt a deep satisfaction knowing that I made her transition to death as peaceful and comfortable as I could have. I had drawn upon my knowledge of ethical standards and professional codes of practice when interacting with senior staff, and this provided me with the framework and courage to advocate for my patient.

As students we can sometimes feel like we don't make a difference or that we don't have the knowledge or experience to advocate and create change, but this experience has shown me otherwise. Nurses are afforded many opportunities to advocate for our patients and I really believe that it is our ethical and professional responsibility to do so.

Student advocacy

As well as acting as advocate for others, you may require an advocate yourself at times during your nursing career. In some circumstances your clinical educator may be able to advocate on your behalf, or your lecturer may be the person who can best represent your interests. Do not hesitate to request this type of support. You should also be aware that there are professional advocates available. A search of websites (e.g. student unions and nurses' associations) will identify some of the services available.

Coaching tips

- Identify the essential human rights that a nurse must respect in order to be a patient advocate.
- Identify your responsibilities as a patient advocate.
- Carefully gather relevant information related to the situation and patient before addressing an issue. Try to stand back and analyse all issues objectively.
- Empower patients to self-advocate rather than taking over (i.e allow patients to ask their own questions of members of the interprofessional healthcare team). Perhaps set the scene so that patients are able to ask their questions or suggest they write their questions down before a consultation.
- Provide patients with information that enables them to make informed decisions.
- Identify the most appropriate person to speak on your behalf should you need an advocate.

MANAGING CONFLICT

Conflict is inevitable and occurs in every workplace and in any relationship. Conflict is difficult and distressing, but it does provide the opportunity for stimulating discussion and for developing your interpersonal skills. Sometimes conflict arises because of a misuse of power, authoritarian tactics or condescension; sometimes it is the result of a misunderstanding or miscommunication; at other times it is simply a personality clash.

In your clinical placements, as in everyday life, you are likely to observe or experience conflict. How effectively you manage the situation will depend on your professional stance, resilience, previous experiences and degree of emotional intelligence. See Chapter 4 for a more detailed discussion of emotional intelligence.

Coaching tips

- When conflict occurs ask yourself if you have done anything to contribute to the situation. Try to be objective and to look at the problem from all sides.
- Keep things in perspective. If the issue is not worth losing sleep over, let it go.
- Confer with the other person in a neutral and private setting (not at the nurses' station or a public place).
- Share your thoughts and feelings. Explain the problem from your perspective: 'I feel …' or 'It seems to me …'

Coaching tips (cont'd)

- Check your understanding. Listen to the other person's perspective. Try to understand the reasons behind the conflict.
- Look for common ground and attempt a compromise. Pursue a good outcome for all involved. If the other person sees you are willing to make some changes to achieve reconciliation, hopefully they will meet you half way.
- Try not to become defensive or use personal attacks.
- Use direct confrontation as a last resort.
- Talk to other students about similar experiences and how they handled them.
- Decide upon a course of action. If a satisfactory compromise cannot be reached, you'll need to make a choice. If you decide to yield to another person's decision, do so without self-pity and resentment. If you decide to stand up for your rights, be aware of relevant policies, the appropriate steps to take and who to speak to (e.g. a mentor, clinical educator, lecturer or counsellor).

Other considerations

Sometimes other factors affect how you view the situation. Consider whether you or the other person involved are either of the following:

- *Fatigued.* Have you been taking care of yourself properly? Could your tiredness be making you unreasonable?
- *Stressed.* Is there something happening in your personal life that is overshadowing your ability to see the situation clearly? Has something happened on the ward to make the other person feel stressed (e.g. a patient death or short staffing)?

DEALING WITH HORIZONTAL VIOLENCE

Although many nurses may not be familiar with the term 'horizontal violence' (or 'workplace bullying'), most have experienced it (and participated in it) at some time during their career. The concept of horizontal violence or bullying has been discussed in the nursing literature for almost two decades. It is defined as nurses covertly or overtly directing their dissatisfaction towards each other and to those less powerful than themselves. This causes harm, disrespects and devalues the worth of that person while denying them their basic human rights (Purpora & Blegan 2012). In the past it was suggested that because nurses were dominated (and, by implication, oppressed) by a patriarchal system headed by doctors, administrators and nurse managers, nurses lower down the hierarchy of power resorted to aggression among themselves. Whether or not this view is still current is debatable. There are many obvious manifestations of horizontal violence, and others that are quite subtle. Some examples include non-verbal behaviours such as ignoring a peer, verbal behaviours such as the sarcastic retort or talking behind someone's back, or physical acts such as pushing someone or slamming of a door (Purpora & Blegan 2012). It is important that you recognise behaviours and organisational structures that may contribute to

STUDENT STORY

They'd sit there for 10 minutes arguing and saying, 'I don't want her, I don't want her'
Elizabeth's story

You'd sit there in handover and the manager of the ward wouldn't allocate you to a registered nurse, so you'd say, 'Who's taking me today?' And they'd sit there for 10 minutes arguing and saying, 'I don't want her, I don't want her'—it was really awful. They didn't want us there and they made it really plain that they just had no interest in students. They'd say, 'I don't have time for students' or 'I'm too busy for students' ... and in front of us, too, so it wasn't even diplomatically done.

I can sort of understand that students are hard work—they take time, they take energy, you're busy already—but you know, we've got to learn somehow. And I really didn't learn in that environment because I felt so unwelcome there I didn't feel comfortable. I felt like if I asked any questions I would just get told to go away.

Each day when I went home and I thought about going back the next day, I just didn't want to. I didn't want to be there. I really questioned whether I wanted to keep going with nursing. I certainly didn't feel like nursing was a good thing in that particular place. And even now I wouldn't want to work in that hospital. And that's almost three years on.

Source: Levett-Jones & Lathlean 2009

workplace bullying and develop strategies for addressing them (Australian Human Rights Commission 2011).

Common examples of horizontal violence (bullying) in nursing include:

- non-verbal innuendo (raising of eyebrows, pulling faces)
- verbal affront (snide remarks, abrupt responses, sarcasm)
- undermining activities (turning away, not being available, exclusion)
- withholding information (about practice or patients)
- sabotage (deliberately setting up a negative situation)
- infighting (bickering with peers)
- scapegoating (attributing all that goes wrong to one individual)
- backstabbing (complaining to others about an individual instead of speaking directly to that individual)
- failure to respect privacy
- broken confidences (Australian Human Rights Commission 2011; Purpora & Blegan 2012).

Horizontal violence is one of the most personally troubling experiences for nurses (Rittenmeyer et al. 2012). Students undertaking a clinical placement have been identified as a group that is especially vulnerable. One reason for this vulnerability is their inexperience, which makes their work subject to scrutiny and criticism. Horizontal violence can cause students significant stress and prevent them from asking questions; they feel as though they don't fit in. Unfortunately, sometimes registered nurses excuse their own behaviour by saying, 'This is how people treated me when I was a student'.

Coaching tips

Understanding the origins and extent of horizontal or workplace violence in nursing will help you realise you are not to blame and that you should not take it personally. Universities and healthcare institutions have policies and procedures for dealing with workplace issues. There are also designated staff for you to turn to for advice and support. It is important that you do not 'suffer in silence' if you observe or experience this type of behaviour. It is also important that you learn how to break the cycle of horizontal violence by confronting the situation rather than trying to ignore it. Confrontation is difficult but often results in the resolution of the bullying behaviour.

Here are some examples of how to confront horizontal violence such as that experienced by Elizabeth (adapted from Griffin 2004):

Action: Dismissive verbal affront such as 'we're just too busy for students'

Response: 'I understand that you may feel like I am an extra burden but if you explain what needs to be done I may actually relieve some of your work.' Or 'If you feel it is too difficult to provide the clinical supervision I need today would you like me to contact the university or my facilitator so they can find another ward for me?'

Action: Non-verbal innuendo (raised eyebrows, face pulling)

Response: 'I sense from your facial expression that there may be something you'd like to say to me. It is fine to speak to me directly.'

Action: Verbal affront (snide remarks or abrupt response)

Response: 'I learn best from people who can give me clear and complete directions and feedback. Could I ask you to be more open with me?'

Action: Backstabbing

Response: 'I don't feel comfortable talking behind his/her back.' (then walk away)

Action: Broken confidences

Response: 'I thought that was shared in confidence.'

Appropriate behaviours for health professionals to prevent horizontal violence (bullying) include:

- respect the privacy of others
- be willing to help when asked
- keep confidences
- work cooperatively despite feelings of dislike
- don't undermine or criticise colleagues
- address colleagues by name, and ask for help and advice when needed
- look colleagues in the eye when having a conversation
- don't be overly inquisitive about other people's lives
- don't engage in conversation about a colleague with another colleague
- stand up for colleagues in conversations when they are not present
- don't exclude people from conversations or social and workplace activities
- don't criticise publicly (adapted from Chaska 2000).

DEALING WITH SEXUAL HARASSMENT

Some authorities contend that the nursing profession has one of the highest rates of sexual harassment (Roche et al. 2010). Sexual harassment is perpetuated by both staff and patients and comes in many guises. Many people tolerate it, some hardly notice it and some find it amusing in small doses and even laugh about it.

Stereotypical images of nurses have played a contributing part in sexual harassment. Media images of nurses are improving, but in the past nurses were often stereotyped as being flirtatious and sometimes sexually promiscuous. Male nurses have been stereotyped too and are sometimes victimised for doing what for years was considered to be 'women's work'.

What one person interprets as sexual harassment may be considered by others as a 'bit of harmless fun'. Harassment can run the gamut from offensive jokes or sexual comments to inappropriate touching. In a study undertaken by Spector et al. (2012), exposure to sexual harassment was experienced by about 25% of nurses worldwide. The majority of these cases are between male patients and female nurses (Spector et al. 2012). Such harassment creates tension for nurses, who must walk a fine line between meeting their professional responsibilities to patients and protecting themselves.

What is sexual harassment?

Sexual harassment is characterised by conduct of a sexual nature that is unwanted and unwelcome to the receiver. Conduct is considered unwelcome when it is neither invited nor solicited and the behaviour is deemed offensive and undesirable. Sexual harassment is defined in the *Sex Discrimination Act 2011* as 'any unwelcome sexual advance, request for sexual favours or conduct of a sexual nature in relation to the person harassed in circumstances where a reasonable person would recognise that the person harassed would be offended, humiliated or intimidated' (Australian Human Rights Commission 2013). In the workplace this is considered to be an unlawful exercise of power.

Harassing behaviours may include:

- verbal sexual advances determined by the recipient as unwelcome
- sexually oriented comments about someone's body, appearance and/or lifestyle
- suggestive comments or jokes
- intrusive questions about one's personal life
- offensive behaviour, such as leering, staring, ridicule or innuendo
- display of offensive visual materials of a sexual nature
- unwelcome physical touching (Australian Human Rights Commission 2013; Lee et al. 2011).

Coaching tips

As a nurse you should be vigilant against sexual harassment. If someone speaks or acts inappropriately towards you this is what you can do:

- Recognise the behaviour.
- Don't blame yourself.
- Keep a diary of what has happened.

Coaching tips (cont'd)

- Tell the person involved that you are uncomfortable with this behaviour and that it offends or scares you. Some people don't realise the effect of their behaviour and are genuinely horrified when told their actions are perceived to be harassing when they thought they were being friendly or amusing. Offenders need to understand that is it not what they intended that matters but how they are perceived.

- Remove yourself from the situation if possible. If a person seems to be targeting you inappropriately, ensure you are never alone with them.

- Give no encouragement. If someone is harassing you, don't respond to them. Do not engage in friendly banter.

- Confide in your clinical educator and/or a colleague if you think someone is harassing you, even if it is only minor pestering.

- Never give your contact details to patients or clinical staff who you do not know well.

- Know your rights and the policies of your educational and healthcare institutions regarding harassment.

- If the situation escalates, report the offender to your educator, mentor or nursing unit manager, who can take appropriate action.

- If a patient speaks to you or touches you inappropriately, challenge the person immediately in a firm, clear, loud voice for other people to hear. If the harassment continues, you can ask to have another nurse stand by in the patient's room, or refuse to care for the patient. *Regardless of what you do, you should report the behaviour to a superior.*

   Remember that sexual harassment is against the law. All educational and healthcare institutions have policies to protect against sexual harassment. Do not tolerate (or perpetuate) it in any form.

TAKING CARE OF YOURSELF

In order to perform at your best and to practise safely it is essential that you care for yourself (Chow & Kalischuk 2008). The NMBA national competency standards (2006, p. 3) stipulates that you should 'consider individual health and wellbeing in relation to being fit for practice'. This is supported by the New Zealand Nurses Organisation (2012). Caring for yourself requires that you proactively adopt healthy lifestyle choices in order to cope with the demands of study, nursing practice, family and social activities. A holistic assessment of your health and wellbeing will help you to identify your needs and any problems that require a change in lifestyle or a review of your ability to practise nursing. Equip yourself with knowledge about health and wellness. Select appropriate strategies and commit to making healthy choices. Caring for yourself and maintaining a work/life balance needs to be a priority.

One area that nursing students often struggle with is maintaining adequate rest and sleep patterns. Fatigue causes many of the same symptoms as those caused by a raised blood alcohol (e.g. being 17 hours sleep-deprived equates with having a 0.05 blood alcohol concentration) (Australian Transport Safety Bureau 2010). This makes you unsafe to practise. If alcohol consumption and fatigue are both present then your symptoms are intensified. The only real cure for tiredness and sleep deprivation is, of course, sleep, with adults needing approximately six to eight hours of quality sleep each 24 hours (Cliff & Horberry 2010).

Coaching tips

- Eat well, get enough rest and sleep, exercise regularly and be kind to yourself. Take a few minutes each day just to reflect and/or meditate. Take this time to renew yourself physically, mentally, emotionally and spiritually. Private time is not a luxury—it is a necessity.
- Keep your body well hydrated, especially during busy shift periods.
- Assess your own health and set up a personal plan that addresses your needs and problems. Seek professional health advice as necessary.
- Ensure you are familiar with the immunisation requirements for practice. Most educational institutions require you to provide evidence of having complied with these requirements before you are authorised to begin your clinical placements.
- Manual handling injuries are one of the most common reasons for nurses' absenteeism. It is vitally important that you learn safe patient-moving techniques and practise these at all times.
- You'll learn a lot about infection control during your studies. Remember that infection control protects both your patients and you and do not forget to use personal protective equipment when appropriate.
- Do not attend you placements if you are unwell. Doing so threatens patient safety because you may be contagious.
- Learn to say no to people who put excessive demands on you. Learn to say yes to activities you really enjoy.
- Develop time-management skills to help you juggle study, friends, family and work. Prioritise and don't leave things to the last minute (the extra stress is just not worth it).
- Implement strategies to lessen the effects of lifestyle and work stressors. Try to eliminate as many of these stressors as possible.
- Practise mind–body therapies as strategies to help restore peace and balance. Learn how to engage in mindfulness meditation, a technique for promoting relaxation and improving focus and clarity of mind. It has been reported to reduce stress, burnout, anxiety and depression, and increase concentration and memory (Wahbeh et al. 2008).

Coaching tips

Coaching tips (cont'd)

- Live a life of gratitude. Regularly reflect on the things you are grateful for—a delicious meal, a walk on the beach, a loving family ... This form of mindfulness creates a positive attitude and sense of harmony.

- Set up support networks with colleagues for clinical placements. These can include childcare support networks, travel groups and study groups.

- Seek professional and academic advice about the impact that a disability may have on your practice or your learning. Most universities have disability officers who can provide support and advice, whether your disability is new, temporary or permanent.

PUTTING WORK AHEAD OF YOUR STUDIES

Clashes between work, study, clinical placements and personal commitments sometimes cause problems for nursing students. Competing commitments can have an impact on your progress and achieving your goals. Thoughtful, advanced planning can prevent later problems. Be mindful that the effects of celebrations, fatigue, travel, illness, alcohol and drugs may lead you to be unproductive and even unsafe on clinical placements, rather than motivated and committed to learn. Consider Kait's story.

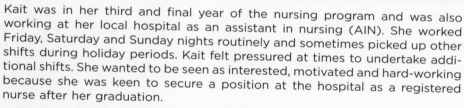

STUDENT STORY
'I worked last night'
Kait's story

Kait was in her third and final year of the nursing program and was also working at her local hospital as an assistant in nursing (AIN). She worked Friday, Saturday and Sunday nights routinely and sometimes picked up other shifts during holiday periods. Kait felt pressured at times to undertake additional shifts. She wanted to be seen as interested, motivated and hard-working because she was keen to secure a position at the hospital as a registered nurse after her graduation.

Even though Kait knew that she would be undertaking a full-time clinical placement in her final semester she did not discuss her roster with her manager. She continued to work her routine hours and added additional shifts when requested.

During the clinical placement, the mentor informed her lecturer that Kait was performing adequately, but because of her evident tiredness it had been decided not to allow her to care for any complex patients, or to undertake any advanced skills. She was not permitted to administer medications and was allocated showering, feeding and bed-making only. Staff felt it was not safe for Kait to perform care commensurate with her educational level. Further discussions between the mentor and the lecturer revealed that Kait had also been sent home the previous day because she was tired. When she admitted she had worked a night shift the previous night, Kait was sent home for safety reasons.

Reflection

Consider the following points in relation to the scenario above:

- Patient safety is the most important issue that needs to be considered. Kait had a responsibility to undertake care to the level of her knowledge in a safe, accountable manner. Her tiredness detracted from her ability to perform safely.

- Kait was required to undertake a compulsory clinical placement as a component of her studies in order to meet her learning goals. As a result of her work commitments she was unable to achieve this outcome during her placement experience.

- Educational institutions have policies that guide student behaviour, both in the classroom and on clinical placements. At Kait's university, her behaviour contravened those policies, and resulted in her failing the placement.

It is important to maintain a work/life balance—this includes your psychological, physical, social and spiritual health. Allow time for study and make thoughtful decisions about where your energy is to be spent. You must be at 'full capacity' on clinical placement to ensure you provide safe nursing care and can learn effectively.

CLINICAL PLACEMENTS AT DISTANT LOCATIONS

If you have the opportunity to undertake a clinical placement in another health service, state/territory or country you are very fortunate. This type of experience will open your eyes to new professional and personal opportunities. However, preparing for a clinical placement at a distance from where you live or study can be very daunting. Just like any other trip, you'll have travel and accommodation details to organise, as well as a host of other practical issues to sort out. Some placements (especially the first placement) require a lengthy timeframe for finalising immunisations and completing police checks before your placement can begin. On top of this there may be social and cultural differences between you, your co-workers and your clients to consider. Undoubtedly policies and procedures will be different from those you are used to, and you won't always have the immediate back-up of academic staff. You also need to consider the learning opportunities available and your specific clinical learning objectives.

Undertaking a clinical placement at a distance can produce a lot of anxiety, which can impact on your learning and your ability to make the most of your experience. We outline here some strategies to help you through what can be a challenging (but exciting) time.

Preparation

- Think about the type of placement that would suit you best, that you can afford and that you are passionate about. It's no good planning a placement with the Royal Flying Doctor Service if you hate flying! Check to see if there is a memorandum of understanding or agreement between the placement and your university.

- Distant placements can be expensive—look at all types of travel and accommodation options and determine whether you or your university is responsible for organising and paying for these. Sharing expenses with fellow students may be possible. In rural areas both food and fuel can also be very expensive. Investigate whether your university, state or territory department of health or nursing organisations provide any financial support.

- Don't leave it to the last minute to get organised. This type of placement can take months to organise.

Coaching tips

Coaching tips (cont'd)

- Preparation requires research. Search on the internet and ask at travel agencies. Most importantly, talk to lecturers and students who have been to the placement institution. Ask lots of questions to get a realistic picture of what to expect.

- You'll need to know about accommodation options, parking, internet and library facilities, what to wear, who your contact person will be, what area you'll be working in, what they expect of you and what you'll be allowed to do.

- Make sure you have a clear and appropriate set of learning objectives.

When you arrive

- Be positive and enthusiastic. Let the people you work with know you are excited to be there and anxious to learn.

- Clarify your student role—in some places you may be expected to just observe; in others to work as part of the team.

- Make sure you discuss your expectations and learning objectives early in the placement.

- Be open to and welcoming of serendipitous learning opportunities.

- Keep a journal or blog—write down the things you encounter and your reactions to it all. It will help you maintain perspective and will be great to look back on.

- Maintain regular contact with your academic support person. Keep the dialogue open and don't be afraid to ask lots of questions. If you are finding it difficult to meet your learning objectives, discuss this early so that an alternative learning plan can be organised.

- Know when and where to seek help and don't hesitate to do so.

- Work to resolve conflict if it arises (for strategies, see previous section).

- Be prepared for things to go wrong. It is unusual for clinical placements to proceed without a hitch. Keep your sense of humour. Try to see something of value in each new problem and challenge.

CLINICAL LEARNING OBJECTIVES

SOMETHING TO THINK ABOUT

Unless you try to do something beyond what you have already mastered, you will never grow.
Ralph Waldo Emerson—essayist, poet and philosopher

When undertaking clinical placements your learning will be both opportunistic and structured. In this section we talk about how clinical objectives help to provide direction and purpose to your learning experience. In some ways a set of clinical objectives is like a well thought out itinerary. It guides your clinical journey, keeps you focused on the most important areas and can be used to communicate what you hope to achieve to others (e.g. clinical educators and mentors) and where your interests lie. Your clinical objectives may be prescribed or you may be required to develop your own in preparation for your placement. Either way they should align with the NMBA national competency standards (2006) and be SMART (Fowler 1998):

S   Specific
M   Measurable
A   Achievable
R   Realistic
T   Timely.

Working towards achievement of a specific set of learning objectives will help you become a safe, effective, competent and confident registered nurse. Your objectives will progressively become more sophisticated as you proceed through your program, and each semester they will build upon and consolidate what you have already learnt.

Coaching tips

When developing your clinical learning objectives you should consider these questions (see also Box 3.3):

- What do you want to learn? (objective)
- Why do you want to learn it? (rationale)
- How are you going to learn it? (strategy)
- How are you going to prove that you have achieved your objective? (evidence)

Box 3.3   An example clinical objective

Objective: To become competent in assessing, interpreting and responding to changes in a person's neurological observations and determining whether they fall within normal parameters for the individual.

Rationale: Neurological assessment is a vital nursing skill and an important indication of a patient's health status.

Strategy: I will research best-practice guidelines regarding neurological assessment, practise the skill in the clinical laboratory on campus and on placement, learn to interpret neurological observations, and ask for feedback from my mentor and educator.

Evidence: When I believe I am competent I will (a) ask my clinical educator to assess my ability to conduct a neurological assessment; and (b) demonstrate my ability to detect alterations in neurological status, to confirm my achievement of this objective.

Developing learning objectives will require you to reflect upon your previous clinical experiences and review your strengths and limitations. Read about reflective practice and the importance of seeking feedback in Chapter 4 before you begin to develop your objectives. You will also need to be self-directed and insightful in order to develop objectives that are meaningful and relevant to your stage of development. Use the NMBA national competency standards as a benchmark to help you analyse what you already know and can do, and where you need to focus, consolidate, develop and improve. Also consider the context of your placement and your scope of practice (see Chapter 1). There is no point in having the objective 'develop knowledge and skills in the management of a central line' if you are a first-year student about to begin a placement in an aged care facility. Remember also that your clinical objectives should focus on the development of knowledge, skills *and* attitudes.

Finally, it is wise to discuss your objectives with your clinical educator or mentor, who will be able to determine if your objectives meet the SMART criteria listed above. It is important to know early on in a placement whether or not your objectives are realistic for your level of experience, and whether you'll be able to achieve your objectives in a particular unit, with a particular patient mix and within a specific timeframe. Don't be surprised if your objectives need to be amended slightly.

STUDENT ASSESSMENT

The clinical learning environment is an important component of formal learning. Assessment of your clinical performance forms an essential part of the teaching–learning process. Ongoing assessment throughout a placement allows you to gain a sense of achievement, to gauge your progress and to appreciate your ability to practise.

Various forms of clinical assessments are used in practice. Some assessments are designed to provide you with ongoing feedback, others determine your competence (perhaps in performing a nursing skill) and some may provide a measure of your skills or knowledge based on a set of criteria (Health Workforce Australia 2014; Levett-Jones et al. 2011). The NMBA *National competency standards for the registered nurse* and the Nursing Council of New Zealand *Competencies for registered nurses* underlie many assessments related to clinical (and on-campus) performance. You may be required to complete a self-appraisal of your performance or undergo peer assessment before your mentor assesses you. Other examples of clinical assessments include:

- undertaking medication administration, with your clinical educator completing a feedback sheet that becomes a critical element of your professional portfolio
- demonstrating and being assessed on non-technical skills such as therapeutic communications skills and clinical reasoning
- attending to a set of nursing care procedures under supervision, which may then be rated according to best-practice guidelines
- collecting data that will form the basis of an assessment item, such as the observation of wound healing.

For some assessments, your university may require you to be assessed by a person who is a qualified assessor (e.g. your clinical educator or an appropriately approved assessor). For other assessments, it may be that the person you are working with (your mentor or preceptor) would be the most appropriate person to assess you. When you inform your facilitator or mentor of your learning objectives at the beginning of the placement, you should also discuss required assessments. Remember that care requirements for patients are always paramount, and your need to complete an assessment must not compromise the health or welfare of a patient. You should also be considerate of staff workloads and other pressures. There are many competing needs in a clinical learning environment, and you should focus on the broader picture rather than your personal needs for assessment only. On some placements there may be situations or issues that make it difficult for you to undertake your required assessments. Examples of these may include constraints imposed by:

- limited opportunities for you to undertake the assessment (e.g. intramuscular injections) in some clinical contexts
- time constraints and the competing demands of others (e.g. patient-care demands)
- a large number of student assessments that need to be undertaken and as a consequence do not allow adequate time for practice or supervision
- some students requiring more time for supervision and assessment than others.

Coaching tips

- Discuss assessment requirements with your facilitator or mentor early in the placement. You may find this facilitates the process and relieves pending anxiety.
- Communicate any difficulties you perceive about meeting the assessment requirements to the appropriate person (this may be the clinical educator, lecturer or registered nurse) as soon as you identify them.
- As with all nursing care, the principles of safe practice must be integrated into your assessment.
- Know and use the NMBA (2006) or Nursing Council of New Zealand (2007) competency standards to inform your practice.
- Take advantage of practice opportunities on campus (such as laboratory and simulation sessions) to ensure you are ready for assessment when on clinical placements.

GIVING AND RECEIVING GIFTS

In this section we focus on giving and receiving gifts, an issue that has the potential to be a boundary violation for nurses (see Chapter 4 for a general discussion of boundary violations). While society views gift-giving as a normal way of showing appreciation, giving or receiving gifts in the context of the nurse–patient relationship has the potential to invoke emotional discomfort and embarrassment, and to compromise a relationship where trust, rapport and the power balance are open to exploitation.

Patients often express their gratitude by giving a small gift at the end of their stay. This type of gift is usually given to one nurse but is accepted on behalf of the team. It may take the form of flowers, chocolates or fruit, which are left at the nurses' station for sharing. Boundary violations can be avoided by declining personal gifts and accepting the gift on behalf of the team.

'Accepting gifts, favours or hospitality may compromise the professional relationship with a health consumer' (Nursing Council of New Zealand 2012, p. 32). At all times nurses must recognise their position and the influence they may have as a professional. Involvement in financial transactions (other than in a contract for the provision of services) and the receipt of anything other than 'token gifts' within professional relationships is likely to compromise the nurse–patient relationship and can be seen as a 'means of securing the nurses' influence or favour' (NMBA 2008b).

In regard to gifts consider:

- the timing of the gift in relation to the patient-care episode (before, during or after care is provided)
- the intent of the gift and any expectation of preferential care being provided as a result of the gift
- the potential consequences of accepting or refusing the gift, such as family responses or any emotional discomfort.

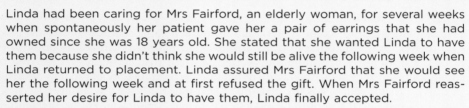

STUDENT STORY
Accepting gifts
Linda's story

Linda had been caring for Mrs Fairford, an elderly woman, for several weeks when spontaneously her patient gave her a pair of earrings that she had owned since she was 18 years old. She stated that she wanted Linda to have them because she didn't think she would still be alive the following week when Linda returned to placement. Linda assured Mrs Fairford that she would see her the following week and at first refused the gift. When Mrs Fairford reasserted her desire for Linda to have them, Linda finally accepted.

Mrs Fairford passed away during Linda's days off and when her family came to collect her belongings they noticed that their mother's earrings were missing. The family demanded that the earrings be found. The patient's room was thoroughly searched, but of course the earrings were not found. The nurse unit manager asked to speak to all staff who had cared for Mrs Fairford. It was during this interview that Linda found out that the earrings she had been given by Mrs Fairford had been reported missing by the family. Mrs Fairford had not informed her family of her decision to give Linda the earrings, nor had Linda told anyone about her gift.

Reflect on this situation. Would you have considered the earrings an appropriate gift? Are they what could be deemed a token gift? Did Linda violate a principle of professional practice? What impact did this gift have on the family and on Linda?

Coaching tips

- Consider carefully whether the gift being offered to you by a patient is an appropriate gift.
- If you do accept a gift, accept it on behalf of the team.
- Seek advice from your mentor or nursing unit manager about any gifts that are offered by a patient or a patient's family.

Gifts of appreciation from students

Students sometimes feel they would like to show their appreciation to staff who have been involved in their learning. When giving a gift, be careful that you do not place a colleague or supervisor in a position where they feel pressured or uncomfortable. Usually, the best way to offer a gift is as a parting gesture. It may be more appropriate if the gift is offered by a group rather than an individual (this, of course, depends on the number of students allocated to the clinical educator or unit). Here are some suggestions for ways to show appreciation (but note that it is not expected that students provide gifts after every placement):

- verbal thanks expressed directly to your mentor and to the manager of the unit
- a card or certificate expressing your appreciation, naming the staff who supported your learning and explaining what you gained from your experience
- a gift such as a pot plant, flowers, a basket of fruit or a box of chocolates
- morning tea for the staff on the last day of the placement.

Accepting thanks

It is equally important to accept appreciation from the nursing staff for your contribution in a professional way. Too often students downplay or minimise their contribution to the work of the nursing team. Minimising words are those that diminish or deprecate the importance of your achievement. Practise responding to compliments and thanks positively, for example, 'Thank you, it was my pleasure'. Don't use words such as 'I only ...', 'It was nothing' or 'I just ...'. If you must be modest, try saying, 'Thank you, I'm pleased with my progress. I really did have a lot of support and guidance from the registered nurses I worked with here.'

VISITORS DURING CLINICAL PLACEMENTS

Clinical placements require a memorandum of understanding or a field agreement between the university and the healthcare facility. These agreements set out requirements, restrictions and conditions for the placement. Students are therefore bound by specific regulations and policies. As a general principle, students are not to receive personal visitors during clinical placement. However, if a personal visit is necessary, you should discuss it in advance with the appropriate person, such as the nurse manager or your facilitator. Facilities usually have policies that guide special circumstances, such as the needs of breastfeeding mothers.

Coaching tips

- Inform your family and friends that it is inappropriate for them to visit you on clinical placement unless it is an emergency.
- Instruct family members about how to contact you in an emergency. Document your placement details (facility, shift, ward and contact number) for urgent contact requirements.
- Ensure your university has your correct contact details (especially emergency contact details).
- If you have unwanted visitors while on a clinical placement, immediately seek assistance from the manager and/or facility security.

USING SUPPLIES FROM THE HEALTHCARE ORGANISATION

Nursing students undertaking clinical placements enter health facilities where resources are calculated and costed for patient care. Those students who help themselves to health facility supplies contribute to costs associated with the health budget. You should also consider what is provided by the facility for staff and what they themselves contribute.

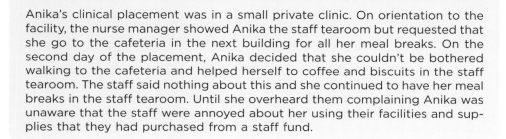

STUDENT STORY
'I didn't realise'
Anika's story

Anika's clinical placement was in a small private clinic. On orientation to the facility, the nurse manager showed Anika the staff tearoom but requested that she go to the cafeteria in the next building for all her meal breaks. On the second day of the placement, Anika decided that she couldn't be bothered walking to the cafeteria and helped herself to coffee and biscuits in the staff tearoom. The staff said nothing about this and she continued to have her meal breaks in the staff tearoom. Until she overheard them complaining Anika was unaware that the staff were annoyed about her using their facilities and supplies that they had purchased from a staff fund.

Not all facilities provide supplies for staff tearooms and you should not assume that food, drink and supplies left in a common tearoom are available for your use. While a cafeteria may be available for staff use, the staff may also contribute to a social club for personal items to support their working environment. These purchases may include:

- tea, coffee, biscuits, milk, sugar and juice
- a filtered water cooler
- a fruit-basket supply
- lunch provisions (bread, butter, spreads, etc.)
- subscriptions to newspapers, magazines or journals.

Apart from tearoom supplies there are also other resources you should think about before helping yourself. For example, letterhead stationery is expensive and students should not use it as notepaper. Nor should you use pre-printed forms (such as medication charts or observation forms) for this purpose.

Similarly, you should ask permission to use the ward photocopier. Think about what it is you are copying, whether you can access the information somewhere else (for instance, from your own computer through internet links or from a library) and the amount of paper that may be used. Also be mindful of copyright laws. Photocopying contributes to the ward or unit budget.

It goes without saying that the health facility is not a place to access supplies for your first-aid kit. Removal of supplies from a facility without permission constitutes theft. Similarly, newspapers and magazines should be left for patients and visitors to read.

PUNCTUALITY AND RELIABILITY

Punctuality and reliability are concepts often discussed in relation to work ethic. We need to consider what our principles are in regard to work, how they will be judged and how they affect others. A lack of punctuality has a significant impact on patient care, the nursing team, their workload and their impression of you as a professional. For example, if you are late for a shift the handover report may need to be repeated for your benefit or, alternatively, you will be required to care for patients without all the relevant information—neither option is satisfactory. Additionally being late or absent may create additional work for staff if they need to notify your university and/or facilitator.

Consider the following story. While it does not specifically focus on the student's role, the principles are nevertheless crucial to your understanding of professionalism.

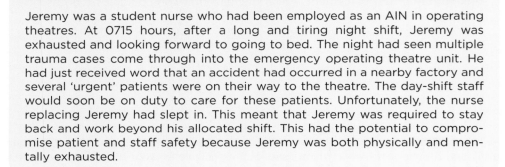

STUDENT STORY
'I'm exhausted'
Jeremy's story

Jeremy was a student nurse who had been employed as an AIN in operating theatres. At 0715 hours, after a long and tiring night shift, Jeremy was exhausted and looking forward to going to bed. The night had seen multiple trauma cases come through into the emergency operating theatre unit. He had just received word that an accident had occurred in a nearby factory and several 'urgent' patients were on their way to the theatre. The day-shift staff would soon be on duty to care for these patients. Unfortunately, the nurse replacing Jeremy had slept in. This meant that Jeremy was required to stay back and work beyond his allocated shift. This had the potential to compromise patient and staff safety because Jeremy was both physically and mentally exhausted.

Coaching tips

- A good work ethic means that you are punctual for all shifts, meetings, appointments and classes.
- Reflect upon your own practices and identify barriers that prevent you from being punctual.
- Be organised and prepare your uniform and clinical placement requirements in advance.
- Notify the appropriate person(s) if an unexpected event occurs that prevents you from being on time.
- For new placements, time the trip to the placement location beforehand (at the same time of the day, if possible).
- Allow plenty of time to get to the ward or unit, as there may be some distance to walk from the car park or public transport stop.

References

ANMC and Nursing Council of New Zealand. A Nurses' Guide to Professional Boundaries. Online. Available: <http://www.anmc.org.au/userfiles/file/PB%20for%20Nurses%20-%20Final%20for%20web%20+PPF%20Watermark%20-%20%20March%202010.pdf>; 2010 Accessed 26.06.10.

Australian Bureau of Statistics. *Media release: 2011 Census reveals one in four Australians is born overseas (No. CO/59)*. Online. Available: <http://www.abs.gov.au/websitedbs/censushome.nsf/home/CO-59?opendocument&navpos=620>; 2012 Accessed 18.02.14.

Australian Commission on Safety and Quality in Health Care. *National safety and quality health service standards*. Online. Available: <http://www.safetyandquality.gov.au/wp-content/uploads/2011/09/NSQHS-Standards-Sept-2012.pdf>; 2014 Accessed 09.01.04.

Australian Human Rights Commission. *Workplace bullying: violence, harassment and bullying fact sheet*. Online. Available: <www.humanrights.gov.au/workplace-bullying-violence-harassment-and-bullying-fact-sheet>; 2011 Accessed 18.01.14.

Australian Human Rights Commission. *Sexual harassment in Australia*. Online. Available: <https://www.humanrights.gov.au/sexual-harassment-australia>; 2013 Accessed 18.01.14.

Australian Transport Safety Bureau. *Roadsafe fatigue. The hidden killer*. Online. Available: <http://www.schools.nsw.edu.au/media/downloads/schoolsweb/leavingschool/eoyc_kit/atsb_fatigue.pdf>; 2010 Accessed 10.01.14.

Braithwaite J, Travaglia JF. An overview of clinical governance policies, practices and initiatives. *Aust Health Rev*. 2008. Online. Available: <http://findarticles.com/p/articles/mi_6800/is_1_32/ai_n28490430>; Accessed 30.12.13.

Brough C. *Language services in Victoria's health system: perspectives on culturally and linguistically diverse consumers*. Melbourne: State Government, Victoria. Published by the Centre for Culture, Ethnicity and Health; 2006. Online. Available: <www.ceh.org.au/resources/resbyceh.html>; Accessed 30.12.13.

Chaska N. *The nursing profession: tomorrow and beyond*. Thousand Oaks: Sage; 2000.

Chow J, Kalischuk RG. Self-care for caring practice: student nurses' perspectives. *IJHC*. 2008;12(3):31-38.

Cliff D, Horberry T. Driving on empty: driver fatigue is dangerous. *QGMJ*. 2010;84-85. Online. Available: <http://www.dme.qld.gov.au/zone_files/QGMJ/safety_and_health_driving_on_empty.pdf>; Accessed 10.01.10.

Cross TL, Basron B, Dennis KW, et al. *Towards a culturally competent system of care* (report). Washington DC: Georgetown University Child Development Center; 1989.

Department of Health Government of Western Australia. *Western Australian clinical governance guidelines*. Information Series No 1.2. Online. Available: <http://www.safetyandquality.health.wa.gov.au/docs/clinical_gov/1.2%20Clinical%20Governance%20Guidelines.pdf>; 2006 Accessed 31.01.14.

Eisenbruch M. *The lens of culture, the lens of health: toward a framework and toolkit for cultural competence*. Sydney: The University of New South Wales; 2004.

Ellis IE, Davey C, Bradford V. Cultural awareness: nurses working with Indigenous Australian people. In: Daly J, Speedy D, Jackson D, eds. *Contexts of Nursing*. 3rd ed. Churchill Livingstone Elsevier; 2010:301-313.

Emanuel L, Berwick D, Conway J, et al. What exactly is patient safety? In: Henriksen K, Battles JB, Keyes MA, et al., eds. *Advances in patient safety: new directions and alternative approaches*. Rockville, MD: Agency for Healthcare Research and Quality; 2008:19-35.

Farrelly T, Lumby B. A best practice approach to cultural competence training. *Aboriginal Isl Health Work J*. 2009;33(5):14-22.

Fernadez A, Seligman H, Quan J, et al. Associations between aspects of culturally competent care and clinical outcomes among patients with diabetes. *Med Care*. 2012;50(9(suppl 2)):S74-S79.

Fowler J, ed. *The handbook of clinical supervision—your questions answered*. Salisbury: Quay Books; 1998.

Garrett PW, Dickson HG, Young L, et al. What do non-English-speaking patients value in acute care? Cultural competency from the patient's perspective: a qualitative study. *Ethn Health*. 2008;13(5):479-496.

Gilligan C, Outram S, Buchanan H. Communicating with people from culturally and linguistically diverse backgrounds. In: Levett-Jones T, ed. *Critical conversations for patient safety: an essential guide for health professionals*. Sydney: Pearson; 2014.

Griffin M. Teaching cognitive rehearsal as a shield for lateral violence: an intervention for newly licensed nurses. *J Contin Educ Nurs*. 2004;35(6):257-264.

Health Workforce Australia. *Clinical training reform. National competency based clinical placement assessment tools*. Online. Available: <http://www.hwa.gov.au/work-programs/clinical-training-reform/clinical-supervision-support-program/national-competency-base>; 2014 Accessed 31.01.14.

Joanna Briggs Institute. *About us*. Online. Available: <http://joannabriggs.org/about.html>; 2013 Accessed 29.01.14.

Johnstone M, Kanitsaki O. Culture, language, and patient safety: making the link. *Int J Qual Health Care*. 2006;18(5):383-388.

Johnstone MJ, Kanitsaki O. Cultural racism, language prejudice and discrimination in hospital contexts: an Australian study. *Diversity in Health and Social Care.* 2008;5:19-30.

Kikuchi JF. Cultural theories of nursing responsive to human needs and values. *J Nurs Scholarsh.* 2005;37(4): 302-307.

Kramer EJ, Ivey S, Ying Y-W, eds. *Immigrant women's health: problems and solutions.* San Francisco: Jossey-Bass; 1998.

Lee S-K, Song J-E, Kim S. Experience and perception of sexual harassment during the clinical practice of Korean nursing students. *Asian Nurs Res.* 2011;5:170-176.

Lehman D, Fenza P, Hollinger-Smith L. *Diversity and cultural competency in health care settings.* Mather LifeWays. n.d.

Leonard M, Graham S, Bonacum D. The human factor: the critical importance of effective teamwork and communication in providing safe care. Sentinel Events Statistics (Joint Commission). *Qual Saf Health Care.* 2004;13:i85-i90.

Levett-Jones T, Gersbach J, Arthur C, et al. Implementing a clinical competency assessment model that promotes critical reflection and ensures nursing graduates' readiness for professional practice. *Nurse Educ Pract.* 2011;1: 64-69.

Levett-Jones T, ed. The relationship between communication and patient safety. *Critical conversations for patient safety: an essential guide for health professionals.* Sydney: Pearson; 2014.

Levett-Jones T, Oates K, MacDonald-Wicks L. The relationship between communication and patient safety. In: Levett-Jones T, ed. *Critical conversations for patient safety: an essential guide for health professionals.* Sydney: Pearson; 2014.

Levett-Jones T, Lathlean J. The 'Ascent to Competence' conceptual framework: an outcome of a study of belongingness. *J Clin Nurs.* 2009;18:2870-2879.

Millenson ML. *Demanding medical evidence.* Chicago: University of Chicago Press; 1997.

Multicultural Health Communication. *Fast facts on language culture and patient safety.* Online. Available: <http://www.multiculturalhealthweek.com/uploads/Fastfacts_on_language_culture_and_patient%20safety.pdf>; 2013 Accessed 10.12.13.

National Health and Medical Research Council. *Cultural competency in health: a guide for policy, partnerships and participation.* Online. Available: <http://www.nhmrc.gov.au/guidelines/publications/hp19-hp26>; 2005 Accessed 10.12.13.

National Patient Safety Foundation. *Patient safety dictionary N–Z.* Online. Available: <http://www.npsf.org/for-healthcare-professionals/resource-center/definitions-and-hot-topics/patient-safety-dictionary-n-z>; 2014 Accessed 31.01.14.

NSW Health. *NSW clinical governance directions statement.* Online. Available: <http://www0.health.nsw.gov.au/resources/quality/pdf/cgudirstat.pdf>; 2005 Accessed 31.01.14.

New Zealand Nurses Organisation. *Standards of professional nursing practice.* Online. Available: <www.nzno.org.nz/resources/nzno_publications>; 2012 Accessed 01.02.14.

Nursing and Midwifery Board of Australia (NMBA). *National competency standards for the registered nurse.* Online. Available: <www.nursingmidwiferyboard.gov.au>; 2006 Accessed 16.01.14.

Nursing and Midwifery Board of Australia (NMBA). *Code of ethics for nurses in Australia.* Online. Available: <www.nursingmidwiferyboard.gov.au>; 2008a Accessed 16.0.14.

Nursing and Midwifery Board of Australia (NMBA). *Code of professional conduct for nurses in Australia.* Online. Available: <www.nursingmidwiferyboard.gov.au>; 2008b Accessed 16.0.14.

Nursing Council of New Zealand. *Competencies for registered nurses.* Online. Available: <http://nursingcouncil.org.nz/Publications/Standards-and-guidelines-for-nurses>; 2007 Accessed 16.01.13.

Nursing Council of New Zealand. *Guidelines for cultural safety, the Treaty of Waitangi and Maori health.* Online. Available: <nursingcouncil.org.nz/Publications/Standards-and-guidelines-for-nurses>; 2011 Accessed 16.01.14.

Nursing Council of New Zealand. *Code of conduct for nurses.* Online. Available: <nursingcouncil.org.nz/Publications/Standards-and-guidelines-for-nurses>; 2012 Accessed 16.01.14.

Paez KA, Allen JK, Beach MC, et al. Physician cultural competence and patient ratings of the patient–physician relationship. *J Gen Intern Med.* 2009;24(2):494-498.

Purpora C, Blegan MA. Horizontal violence and the quality and safety of patient care: a conceptual model. *Nurs Res Pract.* 2012. Online. Available: <www.hindawi.com/journals/nrp/2012/306948/abs>; Accessed 16.01.14.

Reason J. (2000). Human error: models and management. *BMJ,* 320(7237):768-770.

Reason J, Carthey J, de Leval M. Diagnosing 'vulnerable system syndrome': an essential prerequisite to effective risk management. *Qual Health Care.* 2001;10(suppl II):ii21-ii25.

Rittenmeyer L, Huffman D, Block M, et al. A comprehensive systematic review on lateral/horizontal violence in the profession of nursing. *JBI Library of Systematic Reviews.* [S1] 2012;10(42 suppl):S13-S29.

Online. Available: <www.joannabriggslibrary.org/jbilibrary/index.php/jbisrir/article/view/172/159>; Accessed 16.01.14.

Roche M, Diers D, Duffield C, et al. Violence toward nurses, the work environment, and patient outcomes. *J Nurs Scholarsh.* 2010;42(1):13-22.

Schim S, Doorenbos A, Borse N. Cultural competence among Ontario and Michigan healthcare providers. *J Nurs Scholarsh.* 2005;37(4):354-360.

Seaton PL. *Cultural care in nursing: a critical analysis* (PhD thesis). Sydney: University of Technology; 2010. Online. Available: <http://epress.lib.uts.edu.au/research/bitstream/handle/10453/20316/02Whole.pdf ?sequence=4>; Accessed 08.04.14.

Sorensen R, Iedema R. *Managing clinical processes in health services.* Sydney: Churchill Livingstone Elsevier; 2008.

Spector PE, Zhou ZE, Che XX. Nurse exposure to physical and nonphysical violence, bullying, and sexual harassment: a quantitative review. *Int J Nurs Stud.* 2012;51:72-78.

Wahbeh H, Elsas S, Oken B. Mind–body interventions. Applications in neurology. *Neurology.* 2008;70(10): 2321-2328.

Weingart S, Wilson RM. Epidemiology of medical error. *Br Med J.* 2000;320:774-777.

Wilson R, Runciman WB, Gibberd RW, et al. The Quality in Australian Health Care Study. *Med J Aust.* 1995;163:458-471.

Wolff A, Taylor S. An overview of clinical governance. In: Wolff A, Taylor S, eds. *Enhancing patient care: a practical guide to improving quality and safety in hospitals.* Sydney: MJA Books; 2009:1-16.

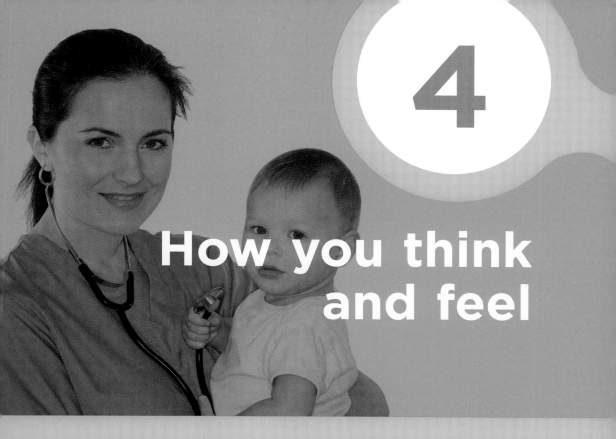

How you think and feel

If one learns from others but does not think, one will be bewildered. If, on the other hand, one thinks but does not learn from others, one will be in peril.

Confucius—Chinese philosopher

INTRODUCTION

In this chapter we challenge you to develop your emotional intelligence, to become a critical thinker and to engage thoughtfully in the clinical reasoning process. We provide an opportunity for you to think consciously and deliberately about your clinical experiences and to reflect on them in ways that are meaningful, memorable and action-oriented. You will also have opportunities to evaluate your strengths and limitations, to consider feedback provided by others, and to develop strategies for improvement. In this chapter we emphasise that the journey of lifelong learning is the responsibility of every nurse and that learning depends upon your ability to be an effective thinker and a reflective practitioner.

CARING

Nurses enter the nursing profession because they care about people and society. You may hear people say 'I was born to be a nurse' or 'I've always wanted to care for others and make a difference in the world'. However, nurses do not have the monopoly on caring. Parents care for their children, teachers care about their students, doctors provide clinical care for their patients, and chaplains provide pastoral care. So what attributes do nurses need to develop in order to become a caring health professional?

It is important to remember that, in nursing, caring manifests in professional behaviours; it is not simply a feeling. Reflect upon encounters that you have had with health professionals—what behaviours demonstrated to you that they cared about you as a person and as a patient?

In nursing, caring is built on a foundation of empathetic accuracy (I understand) and empathetic concern (I care). Effective nurses make conscious choices to behave in ways that are empathetic and that uphold the dignity and inherent human value of each person they care for. This requires you to think about and reflect on another person's experience, values, perspectives and beliefs and to consider how your own attitudes, biases and values affect the person or situation. Self-awareness is integral to empathy and the first step in becoming a caring and competent nurse.

Consider the following questions:

- Nursing is often called the caring profession. Is this how you view nursing?
- Do nurses demonstrate different caring behaviours in different practice contexts? Compare, for example, caring for people in a perioperative setting, in a person's own home or in an aged care facility.
- When observing the nurses you work with, what aspects of their practice would you identify as caring and why?
- Consider how you demonstrate caring in your own practice.
- What would constitute uncaring practices by nurses?
- Consider your personality, beliefs, values, culture, worldview and biases. How do they affect your capacity to be caring towards different people and groups, in particular marginalised groups and those from other cultural backgrounds?

REFLECTIVE PRACTICE

SOMETHING TO THINK ABOUT

The unexamined life is not worth living.
Socrates—Greek philosopher

At the risk of stating the obvious, simply undertaking a clinical placement does not necessarily develop competence—just being there does not guarantee learning. Developing competence involves not only taking action in practice but also learning from practice through reflection. Reflection is intrinsic to learning. It allows nurses to process their experience and explore their understanding of what they are doing, why they are doing it and what impact it has on themselves and others (Boud 1999).

The skill of reflection is pivotal to the development of your clinical knowledge and your clinical reasoning ability. Reflection allows you to consider your personal and professional skills and to identify the need for ongoing development. As a nursing student you should become increasingly aware of your professional values, skills and strengths, as well as the areas that require further development.

While we can and do learn from a wide range of experiences (good and bad), learning is often initiated by painful, difficult, embarrassing or uncomfortable experiences. The adult education theorist Mezirow (1994) calls these experiences 'disorientating dilemmas' and considers them to be a fertile opportunity for developing a critical consciousness. Don't dismiss these challenging times. Reflection is about exploring, questioning, learning and growing through, and as a consequence of, these experiences.

Devoting some time for reflection during and after each clinical placement allows you to plan for future clinical experiences and to develop clear and appropriate objectives for your next placement. Reflecting on your experiences also provides information that you can take to clinical or academic staff for help or guidance in further professional development.

The Nursing and Midwifery Board of Australia (NMBA) *National competency standards for the registered nurse* (2006) specify that competent nurses reflect on practice, feelings and beliefs, and the consequences of these for individuals/groups, to identify personal needs and seek appropriate support.

Keeping a journal

The process of reflection provides the raw data of experiences. In order to use these experiences creatively, and to transform them into knowledge, the additional stage of writing is required. Writing fixes thoughts on paper. As you stare at what you have written, your objectified thinking stares back at you. As you rearrange your writings, you often find you are loosening your imagination by combining various ideas and thoughts. Creative ideas occur during the mechanical process of giving them shape (van Manen 1990). Reflections are the raw materials, but they are turned into knowledge as you write—sometimes you don't know how much you have learnt until you write it down.

Many nursing programs require students to participate in some form of formal written reflection. Students often have to submit a paper-based or electronic journal that describes their reflections about their clinical experience, including application of relevant theory, and their understanding of their experience. Even if this is not a formal requirement at your educational institution, it is certainly wise to keep a personal journal because the reflective writing process allows you to clarify your values, affirm your strengths and identify your learning needs.

Discerning and describing the knowledge, competence and skills that go into day-to-day nursing work allows nurses to understand their work in a more empowering way. This increases nurses' mastery and appreciation of their own work and their ability to provide better care for patients.

SOMETHING TO THINK ABOUT

Observation tells us the fact, reflection the meaning of the fact.
Florence Nightingale—social reformer and nurse (in Baly 1991)

Read Mr Jackson's story, a refection written by a second-year nursing student that illustrates one approach for recording a reflection.

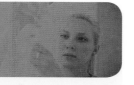

STUDENT STORY

Mr Jackson
Adeola's story

Mr Jackson's story is an example of reflective journal writing and the application of the NMBA *National competency standards for the registered nurse*. Behaviours that reflect an element of the competency standards are followed by the relevant competency number in square brackets.

I was looking after Mr Jackson (pseudonym), a 76-year-old man who was two days post-op following a right hip replacement. As I entered Mr Jackson's room to take his 1000 observations I noticed he was restless and when I spoke to him he did not seem to comprehend my questions, replying inappropriately. I did not recall his confusion being reported at handover [5.2 Uses a range of assessment techniques to collect relevant and accurate data]. *I introduced myself to Mr Jackson and his wife* [9.1 Establishes therapeutic relationships that are goal directed] *and asked whether Mr Jackson had been confused before his hospital admission* [5.2 Uses a range of assessment techniques to collect relevant and accurate data]. *His wife replied that she had never seen him like this before.*

I reassured her and explained [9.2 Communicates effectively with individuals/groups to facilitate provision of care] *that I would take his observations and then consult the RN I was working* with [7.3 Prioritises workload based on the individual's/group's needs, acuity and optimal time for intervention]. *I realised that this situation was beyond my scope of practice* [2.5 Understands and practises within own scope of practice].

I started to consider some of the possible causes for Mr Jackson's confusion. I wondered whether he was in pain, but he did not reply when I asked about his pain. I thought he might have been hypoxic, and when I took his SaO$_2$ it was 88% and his respiratory rate 28. His BP was elevated compared to his pre-op BP; his pulse was rapid, full and bounding. He was afebrile. I checked that his IV fluids were running and his catheter draining. I also checked the wound dressing, which was dry and intact [5.2 Uses a range of assessment techniques to collect relevant and accurate data; 7.1 Effectively manages the nursing care of individual/groups].

I then documented my observations [1.1 Complies with relevant legislation and common law]. *I reassured Mr Jackson and his wife that I would consult with the RN and return* [9.2 Communicates effectively with individual/groups to facilitate provision of care]. *I put the bed rails up* [9.5 Facilitates a physical, psychosocial, cultural and spiritual environment that promotes individual/group safety and security] *before I left the room, as I was concerned for Mr Jackson's safety. I discussed my observations and concerns with the RN* [2.5 Understands and practises within own scope of practice; 10.2 Communicates nursing assessment and decisions to the interdisciplinary healthcare team and other relevant service providers], *who immediately returned with me to review Mr Jackson.*

STUDENT STORY *cont'd*

The RN asked Mr Jackson to point to anywhere it hurt and he touched his head. She checked the IV rate and found it was running at 125 mL/h. When the RN compared the rate to the fluid orders chart, she found it was meant to be running at 84 mL/h. She calculated that the catheter had drained less than 40 mL in four hours. The RN asked Mr Jackson's wife if he was normally so puffy around his eyes and she replied that he wasn't. The RN auscultated his chest and rechecked his SaO_2, this time with an ear probe, as his hands were cold, which she explained could give inaccurate results. The RN explained to Mr Jackson and his wife what she was doing and said she would phone the doctor immediately.

Outside the room the RN explained to me that she suspected hyper-volaemia and possibly electrolyte imbalance and that she was concerned that Mr Jackson would develop pulmonary oedema if he was not treated quickly. She thanked me for bringing Mr Jackson's cognitive changes and abnormal observations to her attention. Review by the doctor and follow-up pathology tests later confirmed the RN's preliminary nursing diagnosis.

I feel I undertook a good but very general assessment of Mr Jackson. However, I realised after watching the RN that I need to develop more focused and comprehensive assessment skills so I can improve my clinical reasoning ability [4.4 Uses appropriate strategies to manage own responses to the professional work environment]. *I also believe that a deeper knowledge base would allow me to analyse and interpret abnormal cues more accurately. In particular, I need an understanding of the potential causes of confusion in elderly patients, and skills and knowl-edge related to fluid status assessment so that I can provide a better standard of care to my patients* [3.1 Identifies the relevance of research to improving individual/group health outcomes]. *It was inspiring to observe an RN who had the experience and clinical reasoning ability to thoroughly and efficiently assess Mr Jackson and establish an accurate nursing diagnosis.*

Coaching tips

There are many resources to help you develop your ability to become a reflective practitioner and your lecturers will probably recommend a specific process. Figure 4.1 is a diagrammatic representation of one model of reflection that we encourage you to use to reflect on your practice and to develop strategies for learning and improvement.

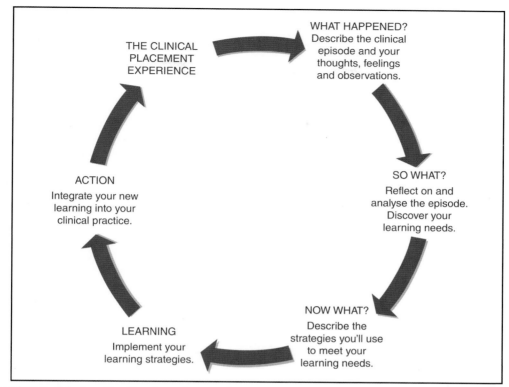

Figure 4.1 A reflective learning cycle
Adapted from Driscoll 2000

REALITY CHECK AND SEEKING FEEDBACK

So far the focus in this book has been on the clinical environment and your place in it. Now it's time to turn the focus completely onto you, by asking you to address the following questions:

- How do I see myself?
- How do others see me?

This is not a once-only activity, but rather a lifelong process of personal and professional development. This 'reality check' is pivotal to your ongoing growth and improvement and is a process that you'll find invaluable to your career success.

How do I see myself?

To answer this question you should begin by assessing and listing your skills and attributes (clinical, interpersonal and others) and identifying your strengths and limitations. Skills are acquired abilities. Attributes may be acquired or intrinsic. There are three main types of skills and attributes:

- technical or clinical skills, such as those involved in safely administering medications or undertaking complex wound dressing procedures
- interpersonal and non-technical skills, which include communication, clinical reasoning, teamwork and empathy (among others)

- personal attributes, such as integrity, adaptability, motivation, resilience, cultural aware-ness and problem-solving ability.

Take some time to reflect on your skills and consider areas in which you excel and those that require further development. Identifying gaps or limitations is just as important as acknowledging your strengths.

How do others see me?

Once you have completed your self-assessment you should validate it by seeking feedback from others. You can obtain this feedback from managers, employers, educators, clinicians and fellow students. Performance appraisals and informal feedback are invaluable to under-standing how others perceive you. Asking for feedback is not always easy, but your success depends on your openness to different perspectives. It involves listening and accepting posi-tive and negative feedback and acknowledging the areas in which change and improvement are needed. Seeking advice about new skills that you require and strategies to develop them are also essential.

Now compare the skills and attributes you identified with the feedback from others. Are there any discrepancies? Did others recognise skills and attributes that you were not aware of but can now build on? Were limitations identified that you were not aware of?

SOMETHING TO THINK ABOUT

If life is to have meaning, the extent to which you know yourself is the most important work that you will ever do.

Source: Crow 2000, p. 33

Coaching tips

It is your right (and responsibility) as a student to seek ongoing and regular feedback about your performance. Most educational institutions have a formal process to ensure this occurs. However, you should still seek informal feedback regularly. Make time for regular performance conversations. Ask for specific concrete feedback about your skills, attributes, strengths and limitations and use the feedback as a springboard to success.

Receiving formal feedback should be a positive experience and should not display any hidden agendas, such as the discussion of any previously unmentioned problems. All problem areas should be dealt with when they occur and not stored up to be revealed only at a performance review. You deserve regular formative feedback throughout your placement and opportunities to improve.

Grievance procedures are available if disagreements are unable to be resolved between you and your assessor; you should consult your educational policies for guidance. Conflict and confusion, if they arise, should be dealt with constructively and sensitively.

EMOTIONAL INTELLIGENCE

To survive and succeed in nursing you need to develop not only technical skills and knowledge but also emotional intelligence. Emotional intelligence is the ability to identify and manage the emotions of one's self and of others. Some argue that emotional intelligence is a determining factor in achieving competence and a more accurate predictor of success than intellectual ability (Goleman 1998). Emotional intelligence is a term that encompasses the human skills of self-awareness, self-control and adeptness in relationships, all of which are recognised as being central to effective nursing practice. Emotionally intelligent individuals excel in human relationships, show marked leadership skills, perform well at work, and are resilient (Goleman 1996). Emotional intelligence also includes persistence, the ability to motivate oneself and altruism. At the root of altruism lies empathy and the ability to read emotions in others, which forms the basis of therapeutic relationships (see Chapter 5). If empathy is limited or lacking, there is no sense of another's need or despair and no care or compassion.

A wealth of literature supports the view that therapeutic relationships between nurses and patients are correlated with positive patient outcomes. As nursing is a 'significant, therapeutic interpersonal process' (Peplau 1952, p. 16), nursing students must develop competence in dealing with their own and others' emotions. The emotional state of the patient/client is often heightened during illness, and nurses should be equipped to respond with empathy and genuine concern. It is important to understand that people who are experiencing illness, stress, anger, pain, fear or frustration may react in different ways. Some will become quiet and withdrawn, others angry or aggressive. While the former seems easier to manage, the nurse still requires skills in therapeutic engagement to provide support and care. By contrast, anger and verbal abuse from a patient or carer may adversely influence a nurse's perception of a patient (O'Grady et al. 2012) While it is natural to want to protect oneself by emotionally withdrawing or angrily responding to a threatening or verbally abusive patient, it is necessary to overcome the emotional impact and still address the patient's needs, conflicts and stressors. Consider the following example and how you might feel if confronted with the situation recounted by this nurse:

> My patient had cancer and refused treatment. As she was found to be able to make that decision we were treating her palliatively. Her daughter said that I was an incompetent f***** who was unable to f***** do anything f***** right and would I go get some other stupid nurse who might at least want to keep patients alive. Then she said she was going to take her mother out of this f***** place.
>
> (Stone 2009, p. 180)

Coaching tips

In dealing with these types of situations it is important to first understand one's own emotional reaction. Then try to moderate your initial response and begin to understand the person's emotional reaction and the reason for it. This may sound easy, but it isn't. Nurses are only human and in most cases when they feel wounded by a patient's verbal aggression or swearing, there is a strong sense of hurt stemming from the discrepancy between the care the nurse perceives they have invested in the patient and the patient's or carer's lack of appreciation of that care (Stone 2009). However, the core of emotional intelligence is empathy—the

Coaching tips (cont'd)

capacity to understand another person's subjective experience from within that person's frame of reference (Castillo et al. 2013). It includes the inclination to invest therapeutic effort by putting into action appropriate and constructive responses, even when the patient's behaviour has been emotionally damaging, and even when one's natural reaction is to withdraw or to become defensive. Emotional intelligence is enhanced through a deliberate process of thoughtful, honest reflection and open dialogue.

There may also be times when you need to use resilience and emotional intelligence when dealing with challenging nursing colleagues. Students who have highly developed emotional intelligence are more likely to view negative and unreceptive staff with a degree of dispassion, rather than taking the staff's rebuttal as a personal affront. They can also accept that 'personality clashes' are an inevitable facet of working life.

STUDENT STORY

'It's learning how to interact with people and deal with people that makes a big difference'
Nadeem's story

It's just a case of just getting on with it. I've learnt over the years you don't take their rejection personally; often it's not a personal thing against you. It's just that some nurses have obviously got issues or something going on in their lives that's making them react the way they react. I don't take it personally. I just think, 'Well okay, we'll just leave that one well enough alone for now' … I think it's learning how to interact with people and deal with people that makes a big difference. It's probably something I would not have been able to do when I started my degree.

Source: Levett-Jones 2007, p. 196

CRITICAL THINKING AND CLINICAL REASONING

SOMETHING TO THINK ABOUT

Thinking leads man to knowledge. He may see and hear, and read and learn whatever he pleases, and as much as he pleases; he will never know anything of it, except that which he has thought over, that which by thinking he has made the property of his own mind.
Johann Heinrich Pestalozzi—Swiss educational reformer

Critical thinking

In nursing, as in healthcare, terms such as critical thinking, clinical reasoning, clinical judgement, diagnostic reasoning and clinical decision making are often used interchangeably (Levett-Jones 2013). There are various definitions of the terms and little consensus on their meaning. In this section we clarify these terms with a particular focus on critical thinking and clinical reasoning.

Critical thinking is a complex collection of cognitive skills and affective habits of the mind. It has been described as the process of analysing and assessing thinking with a view to improving it (Paul & Elder 2007). To become a professional nurse requires that you learn to think like a nurse. This includes an understanding of the knowledge, ideas, concepts and theories of nursing, and the development of intellectual capacities, in order to become a disciplined, self-directed, critical thinker (Paul & Elder 2007).

Critical thinking is the intellectual process of applying skilful reasoning as a guide to belief or action. It is the ability to think in a systematic and logical manner and with openness. Critical thinking also requires the ability to question and reflect on practice.

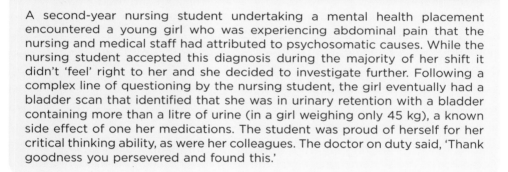

STUDENT STORY
'It just didn't feel right'
Madeline's story

A second-year nursing student undertaking a mental health placement encountered a young girl who was experiencing abdominal pain that the nursing and medical staff had attributed to psychosomatic causes. While the nursing student accepted this diagnosis during the majority of her shift it didn't 'feel' right to her and she decided to investigate further. Following a complex line of questioning by the nursing student, the girl eventually had a bladder scan that identified that she was in urinary retention with a bladder containing more than a litre of urine (in a girl weighing only 45 kg), a known side effect of one her medications. The student was proud of herself for her critical thinking ability, as were her colleagues. The doctor on duty said, 'Thank goodness you persevered and found this.'

Coaching tips

Strive to be a reflective critical thinker. Nursing students who are critical thinkers value and adhere to intellectual standards. They strive to be clear, accurate, precise, logical, complete, significant and fair when they listen, speak, read and write. Critical thinkers think deeply and broadly (Paul & Elder 2007). As nurses, we want to eliminate irrelevant, inconsistent and illogical thoughts as we reason about client care. Incorporating reflection into our practice enhances critical thinking (Freshwater 2008). Nurses use language to clearly communicate in-depth information that is significant to nursing care. They are not focused on the trivial or irrelevant. Nurses who are critical thinkers hold all their views and reasoning to these standards so that the quality of their thinking improves over time. Critical thinking includes a commitment to develop and maintain habits of mind (see Table 4.1), the competent use of thinking skills, engaging in reflective practice and the ability to effectively engage in clinical reasoning.

Table 4.1 **Critical thinking—habits of mind**

Habit	Description	Example
Confidence	Assurance of one's thinking abilities	My thinking was on track. I reconsidered and still thought I'd made the right decision. I knew my conclusion was well-founded.
Contextual perspective	Considerate of the whole situation, including relationships, background, situation and environment	I took in the whole picture. I was mindful of the situation. I considered other possibilities. I considered the circumstances.
Creativity	Intellectual inquisitiveness used to generate, discover or restructure ideas; the ability to imagine alternatives	I let my imagination go. I thought 'outside of the box'. I tried to be visionary.
Flexibility	Capacity to adapt, accommodate, modify or change thoughts, ideas and behaviours	I moved away from traditional thinking. I redefined the situation and started again. I questioned what I was thinking and tried a new approach. I adapted to the new situation.
Inquisitiveness	Eagerness to learn by seeking knowledge and understanding through observation and thoughtful questioning in order to explore possibilities and alternatives	I burned with curiosity. I needed to know more. My mind was racing with questions. I was so interested.
Intellectual integrity	Seeking the truth through sincere, honest processes, even if the results are contrary to one's assumptions or beliefs	Although it went against everything I believed, I needed to get to the truth. I questioned my biases and assumptions. I examined my thinking. I was not satisfied with my original conclusion.
Intuition	Insightful patterns of knowing brought about by previous experience and pattern recognition	I had a hunch. While I couldn't say why, I knew from the previous time this happened that …
Open-mindedness	Receptiveness to divergent views and sensitivity to one's biases, preconceptions, assumptions and stereotypes	I tried not to judge. I tried to be open to new ideas. I tried to be objective. I listened to other perspectives.

Table 4.1 *cont'd*

Habit	Description	Example
Perseverance	Pursuit of learning and determination to overcome obstacles	I was determined to find out. I would not accept that for an answer. I was persistent.
Reflective	Contemplation of assumptions, thinking and action for the purpose of deeper understanding and self-evaluation	I pondered my reactions, what I had done and thought. I wondered what I could have or should have done differently. I considered what I would do differently next time. I considered how this would influence my future practice.

Adapted from Scheffer & Rubenfeld 2000 and Rubenfeld & Scheffer 2006

SOMETHING TO THINK ABOUT

Thinking like a nurse is a form of engaged moral reasoning. Educational practices must help students engage with patients with a deep concern for their well-being. Clinical reasoning must arise from this engaged, concerned stance, always in relation to a particular patient and situation and informed by generalised knowledge and rational processes, but not as an objective, detached exercise.

Source: Tanner 2006, p. 209

Clinical reasoning

Clinical reasoning is defined as the way clinicians critically think about the problems they deal with in clinical practice (Elstein & Bordage 1991). It involves clinical judgements (deciding what is wrong with a patient) and clinical decision making (deciding what to do). Levett-Jones and Hoffman (2013) define clinical reasoning as a logical process by which nurses (and other clinicians):

- collect cues
- process the information
- come to an understanding of a patient's problem or situation
- plan and implement interventions
- evaluate outcomes
- reflect on and learn from the process.

Clinical reasoning is not a linear process but can be conceptualised as a cycle of linked clinical encounters. In Figure 4.2 the cycle begins at 1200 hours and moves in a clockwise

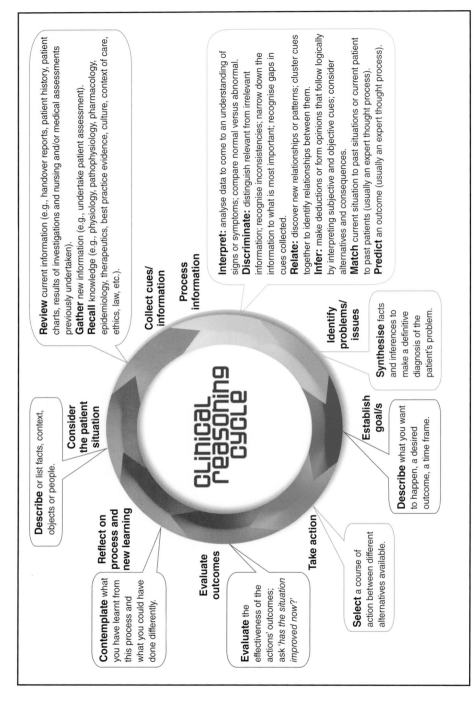

Figure 4.2 The clinical reasoning process with descriptors
Source: Levett-Jones & Hoffman 2013

direction. The circle represents the ongoing and cyclical nature of clinical encounters and the importance of evaluation and reflection. There are eight main steps or phases in the clinical reasoning cycle. However, the distinctions between the phases are not clear-cut. While clinical reasoning can be broken down into the steps of *look, collect, process, decide, plan, act, evaluate* and *reflect*, in reality the phases merge and the boundaries between them are often blurred. While each phase is presented as a separate and distinct element in Figure 4.2, clinical reasoning is a dynamic process and nurses often combine one or more phases or move back and forth between them before reaching a decision, taking action and evaluating outcomes (Levett-Jones et al. 2013). See Figure 4.3 for an example of how the clinical reasoning cycle can be applied to your learning—this clinical reasoning example was provided by a first-year nursing student from CQUniversity.

Why do nursing students need to learn how to engage in clinical reasoning?

Clinical reasoning errors have been identified as the root cause of more than 57% of adverse patient outcomes (Wilson et al. 1995); this includes a failure to collect, interpret and act on clinical data. 'Failure to rescue', defined as the mortality of patients who experience a hospital-acquired complication, is directly related to nurses' clinical reasoning skills. Health professionals poor clinical reasoning skills often fail to detect impending patient deterioration, which results in this 'failure to rescue' (Aiken et al. 2003).

Clinical reasoning is an essential component of competence (Banning 2008). The NMBA *National competency standards for the registered nurse* (2006) refer to the importance of clinical reasoning in Domain 3 (Provision and Coordination of Care) and explicitly outline the importance of the following elements when undertaking patient care:

- conducting a comprehensive and systematic nursing assessment
- planning nursing care in consultation with individuals/groups, significant others and the interdisciplinary healthcare team
- providing comprehensive, safe and effective evidence-based nursing care to achieve identified individual/group health outcomes
- evaluating progress towards expected individual/group health outcomes in consultation with individuals/groups, significant others and the interdisciplinary healthcare team.

Beginning nurses do not always possess an adequate level of clinical reasoning ability. The reasons for this are multidimensional but include the difficulties novice nurses encounter when differentiating between a clinical problem that needs immediate attention and one that is less acute, and a tendency to make errors in time-sensitive situations where there is a large amount of complex data to process. By contrast, experienced nurses engage in multiple clinical reasoning episodes for each patient in their care. An experienced nurse may enter a room and immediately collect significant data, draw conclusions and initiate appropriate management. As a result of their knowledge, skills and experience, expert nurses may appear to perform these processes in a way that seems almost automatic or instinctive; and they often find it difficult to verbalise their thinking and explain cognitive processes that seem tacit and implicit (Levett-Jones & Hoffman 2013).

Hoffman's (2007) research described how beginning and experienced nurses make decisions in the real world of practice and the thinking strategies used while caring for patients. These thinking strategies included: describing the patient situation; collecting new patient information; reviewing information; relating information; recalling knowledge; interpreting information; making inferences; discriminating between relevant and irrelevant information; matching and predicting information; synthesising information to diagnose or identify

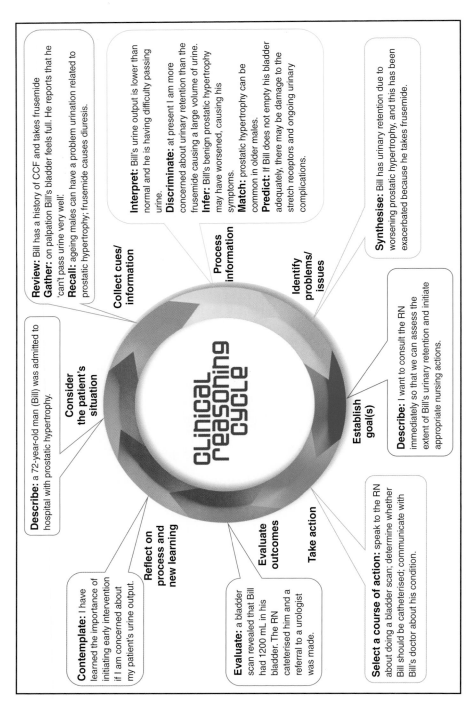

Figure 4.3 The clinical reasoning process applied to a clinical scenario
Source: An example of how the CR cycle can be applied to your learning – this clinical reasoning example was provided by a first year student from CQUniversity.

a problem; establishing goals; choosing a course of action; and evaluating outcomes. This body of research was subsequently used to create the clinical reasoning cycle (Levett-Jones & Hoffman 2013). Hoffman's study found that expert nurses collected more cues than novice nurses and from a wider range of information than novices. Experts also related more cues together than novices and were better able to predict what may happen to a patient. They often practised proactively, collecting a wide range of cues to identify and prevent possible patient complications. In contrast, beginning nurses' practice was more reactive, searching for patient cues and information once they had actually identified a patient problem (Hoffman 2007). These differences have implications for patient safety, with beginning nurses often detecting problems later than expert nurses.

In order for students to learn to manage complex clinical situations and to identify 'at-risk' patients, teaching and learning approaches are needed that make these seemingly automatic thinking processes explicit and clear. Therefore, it is essential that students learn the process and steps of clinical reasoning. Learning to reason effectively does not happen serendipitously, nor does it occur just through observation of expert nurses in practice. Clinical reasoning requires a different approach from that used when learning more routine nursing procedures. It requires a structured educational model and active engagement in deliberate practice, as well as reflection on activities designed to improve performance (Ericsson et al. 2007).

Prior to engaging in clinical reasoning it is important to understand that flawed preconceptions, prejudices and incorrect assumptions—such as 'most Indigenous people are alcoholics', 'women tend to have a lower pain threshold than men' and 'elderly people often have dementia'—will negatively influence one's reasoning ability (Alfaro-LeFevre 2013). McCarthy (2003) identified how nurses' personal philosophies about ageing influence how they manage older hospitalised patients who experience symptoms of delirium. In a study by McCaffery et al. (2000), nurses' opinions of their patients and their personal beliefs about pain significantly influenced the quality of their pain assessment and management. Croskerry (2003) also identified that patients from minority groups and those from culturally and linguistically diverse backgrounds are too often blamed for their illness rather than using clinical reasoning skills to determine the real cause of the health problem. Therefore, in preparation for clinical reasoning it is important that you reflect on and question your assumptions and prejudices; failure to do so may negatively impact on your clinical reasoning ability and, consequently, patient outcomes (Levett-Jones 2013).

Coaching tips

Clinical reasoning and critical thinking takes practice. Multiple opportunities for 'cognitive rehearsal' (a method of mentally processing and practising effective responses to specific situations in order to develop and integrate effective skills into one's repertoire of behaviours) are required for you to learn and effectively apply clinical reasoning in practice.

You need to actively engage in clinical reasoning independently as well as in the learning opportunities provided on campus (such as simulation sessions and tutorials). You also need to make the most of the opportunities provided for the development and application of clinical reasoning skills when you undertake clinical

Coaching tips

Coaching tips (cont'd)

placements. Ask the registered nurses you work with to *think aloud*. Although experienced nurses often find it difficult to verbalise their thinking and explain their cognitive processes you can help by asking questions based upon your understanding of the clinical reasoning process. For example, ask your mentor which information (cues) they collect about specific patients and how they interpret those cues to come to a nursing diagnosis. Or ask them to predict what might happen to a patient if different courses of action were taken.

Higher order questions are particularly helpful in developing your critical thinking skills and developing clinical reasoning ability. These include questions that cause you to analyse, synthesise, cluster cues, match patterns in the cues collected, make inferences, evaluate and apply. Ask yourself (or, better still, prompt your clinical educator or mentor to ask) the following types of questions:

- What is the patient's potential nursing diagnosis?
- What cues would you collect to confirm this diagnosis?
- What are your immediate nursing actions in this situation?
- What might happen if you did nothing in this situation?
- How could you tell if your actions improved the situation for this patient?

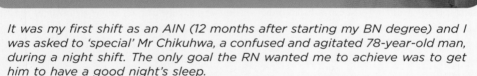

STUDENT STORY
'I was beginning to think like a nurse'
Jaclyn's story

It was my first shift as an AIN (12 months after starting my BN degree) and I was asked to 'special' Mr Chikuhwa, a confused and agitated 78-year-old man, during a night shift. The only goal the RN wanted me to achieve was to get him to have a good night's sleep.

I went and did Mr Chikuhwa's vital signs. He was hypertensive, tachycardic, tachypnoeic and afebrile. At around 2300 hours he wanted to go to the toilet. He was quietly groaning while passing urine, and when I put him back to bed I asked him if he was experiencing any pain; he said he was. I asked Mr Chikuhwa to rate his pain, to which he responded with a nine. I observed his medication chart and noticed he was supposed to have had paracetamol two hours previously.

I approached the RN on duty and updated her with information I had gathered about Mr Chikuhwa. She administered paracetamol and then said, 'Okay, you've brought the patient's situation to my attention, what should you be doing at this point?'. I froze. I eventually responded with, 'Well, there isn't a fluid balance chart in place so I am unable to determine Mr Chikuhwa's fluid input–output to work out if he is in a positive or negative status.'

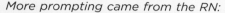

STUDENT STORY *cont'd*

More prompting came from the RN:

'What are you going to do about that, then?'

'Put one in place,' I responded.

'So what would your next action be?' she asked.

'Perhaps attempt to get a urine sample and test that to see if any bacteria or protein is present?' I suggested.

So the next time Mr Chikuhwa went to the toilet I did a dipstick to test his urine—the result was normal and I was stumped. I honestly thought he must have had a urinary tract infection. But I gathered my thoughts about the next possible step for Mr Chikuhwa.

I did his vital signs again at 0400; they were the same as before. I took him to the toilet and again I could hear him groaning and straining to pass urine. I put him back to bed and approached the RN again, saying 'I think we should do a bladder scan on him' and I gave my rationale. So the RN did a bladder scan and was amazed that Mr Chikuhwa had 965 mL in his bladder! My mind was trying to remember how much a bladder can 'normally' hold. I was certain it was 300–350 mL and the RN confirmed this. At 0515 Mr Chikuhwa was catheterised. This poor man had urinary retention and I was amazed that cues weren't picked up prior to me getting there. The RN said, 'Thank you. You did a wonderful job tonight!'. I was walking on cloud nine and so proud of myself. So the moral is … I thought I knew nothing until this incident occurred. I wasn't sure I was retaining a lot of what I had been learning at uni, but it was like a light-bulb moment that just went off. I found myself thinking about the clinical reasoning cycle often during the shift, and I can honestly say that I can now see the significance of it and the biggest thing to come out of this: I was beginning to think like a nurse!

ETHICAL DILEMMAS IN NURSING

SOMETHING TO THINK ABOUT

You should not decide until you have heard what both have to say.
Aristophanes—Greek playwright

What is ethics and why do nurses need to understand it?

The way we practise as health professionals is subject to professional and ethical codes (Johnstone 2009; NMBA 2008). Ethics is often defined as the philosophical study of right or wrong action (Dahnke & Dreher 2006). This does not mean that ethics is of concern to philosophers alone, however. All human beings have pondered questions of right and wrong from time to time. It is essential for nurses to understand ethics because in their day-to-day professional work they frequently encounter ethical questions and dilemmas related to human values and dignity, end-of-life decision making, autonomy and justice, for example. A clear understanding of ethics helps nurses to interpret these difficult situations and to identify possible courses of action (Dahnke & Dreher 2006).

Examples of ethical principles

Principles are standards that make up an ethical system. The following ethical principles underpin health professionals' practice:

- **autonomy:** the ability to make free choices about oneself and one's life, to be self-governing (this principle is at the heart of informed consent)
- **beneficence:** to do good, and the obligation to act for the benefit of others
- **non-maleficence:** to avoid doing harm
- **justice:** fairness and the equal distribution of benefits and burdens
- **veracity:** honestly, truthfulness and integrity.

What is an ethical dilemma?

A 'dilemma' is defined as a problem where there is a choice to be made between options that seem equally unfavourable. An ethical dilemma is even more complex. There may be conflicting ethical principles that apply equally in a given situation, and neither can be chosen without violating the other.

Consider the case of a nurse who accepts the ethical principle that demands sanctity of life but who also accepts the ethical principle of non-maleficence, which demands that people should be spared intolerable suffering. Imagine this nurse caring for a person who is terminally ill and suffering intolerable and intractable pain. In this situation, if the nurse accepts the sanctity-of-life principle, he or she would not be able to sanction the administration of the large and potentially lethal doses of narcotics that may be required to alleviate the patient's pain. However, if the principle of non-maleficence were followed, the nurse might be required to administer potentially lethal doses of narcotics, even though this would probably hasten the patient's death.

In this situation the nurse is confronted with a profound ethical dilemma. To uphold the sanctity-of-life principle would violate the principle of non-maleficence, and to uphold the principle of non-maleficence might violate the sanctity-of-life principle. In everyday nursing practice the nurse would be guided by both principles; however, the ultimate question for the nurse in this situation is 'Which ethical principle should I choose?' (Johnstone 2009).

In another situation, a nurse was caring for an 80-year-old Chinese woman who had been diagnosed with metastatic cancer. The doctor and nurses believed that the patient had the right to be told her prognosis. However, the patient's family did not want her to be told and wanted to make any health-related decisions themselves. The nurses and doctors were caught between a duty to tell the patient the truth (veracity) to promote her right to autonomy, and a duty to respect the family's wishes. Further complicating this dilemma is that ethics is often mediated by the individual's background culture. For example, many traditional Chinese families value collective decision making, and this preference must be taken into account in health-related decisions. Health professionals' ethical beliefs therefore need to be viewed in parallel with the person's cultural beliefs and practices. See Chapter 3 for a more detailed discussion of culturally competent practice.

Ethics is a complex concept that you will undoubtedly study in your nursing program. You would be wise to consider and reflect upon ethical situations as they arise in your nursing practice, being guided by ethical principles and the NMBA *Code of ethics for nurses in Australia* (2008) or the New Zealand Nurses' Organisation's *Code of ethics* (2010). Keep in mind, however, that learning about ethics will make it more likely that you will encounter ethical issues in your practice. Palmer (2013) suggests this is because nurses become increasingly likely to 'see' the ethical dimensions of practice and that their perceptions fundamentally change as a result of such education. But being more attuned and aware of the ethical dimensions of practice is just the beginning. Competent nurses also need to apply that knowledge to practice. This can be difficult because each situation is unique and clinicians need to determine how the generalities of ethical codes actually do or do not apply (Palmer 2013).

What is moral distress?

Ethical dilemmas, when they arise, can cause moral distress and emotional turmoil. Moral distress is the stress associated with the moral dimensions of practice (Varcoe et al. 2012) due to inconsistency between one's values and one's actions. For example, a health professional may recognise the vulnerability of their patients and care about their wellbeing, yet be reticent to speak up and fearful of conflict (Ray 2006); while at the same time be committed to the values of their professional codes of ethics. This is likely to result in moral distress (Elkovich & Barrett 2014).

Coaching tips

- Reflect on ethical dilemmas that have caused you moral distress in the past. What action, if any, did you take in the situation? Who did you or could you have spoken to about the situation? What did you learn from the ethical dilemma that may improve your future practice?
- Always remember that in these situations you are not alone. By communicating with your colleagues, clinical educator and/or mentor you will find the support and guidance you need to manage and learn from the ethical dilemmas you encounter.

CROSSING THE LINE

As a nursing student you will have many roles apart from that of a health professional. These roles may include neighbour, family member, friend and community member. There may be times when the boundaries between your roles seem to blur. An example of this is when you become aware that one of the patients on your ward is someone you know. The NMBA and the New Zealand Nursing Council have developed guidelines to inform nurses of expectations related to professional boundaries (Nursing Council of New Zealand 2012; NMBA 2010). Each health facility also has a code of conduct that should be referred to in relation to boundaries of practice.

What are boundaries?

Boundaries are limits to appropriate behaviour in our personal and professional relationships. In Australia, phrases such as 'crossing over the line' and 'overstepping the mark' are commonly used to describe inappropriate behaviour. Professional boundaries in nursing are defined as limits that protect the space between the professional's power and the patient's vulnerability (Nursing Council of New Zealand 2012; NMBA 2010).

What purpose do boundaries serve?

Maintaining appropriate boundaries in a nurse–patient relationship facilitates therapeutic practice and results in safe and effective care. Nurses and nursing students may be too cold, distant or formal and not caring enough to be helpful. Conversely, they may be overly involved, too interested, or physically invasive. The creation of even a platonic relationship with a patient during a therapeutic encounter increases patient vulnerability, as does caring for a patient who you know from work, university or your community. There is a need to ensure the nurse–patient relationship is always conducted with the sole intent of benefiting the patient. Knowing the difference between a professional and a personal relationship, being a friend versus being friendly, and being able to recognise boundaries between these may seem like common sense. However, recognition of these boundaries requires knowledge and skills that are acquired through time, experience and by working within professional codes of conduct. Consider the following situation.

STUDENT STORY
'I trusted you'
Jenny's story

A student nurse (James) was undertaking a clinical placement in a mental health unit when a fellow student (Jenny) was admitted following her attempted suicide. James did not know Jenny well but decided to call in and say hello to her. During the course of the next week James spent a lot of time with Jenny, believing his support to be therapeutic. Jenny opened up to him, sharing many details about her life. James also began to disclose his own experiences of depression and how it was managed.

On return to university James happened to mention to some fellow students 'in confidence' that Jenny had been admitted to the mental health unit where he had undertaken his clinical placement. He hoped they would be sensitive to the situation and supportive when Jenny returned to university. As often happens, 'news' spread and Jenny found out. She was devastated that James had broken her trust, even more so because she had shared so many sensitive details about her life with him. Jenny decided not to return to university. James was reported for misconduct.

Consider the implications of the above situation. The outcome could have been avoided if James had recognised and understood the professional boundaries of practice.

As a student you may not have enough experience to guide your decisions and it is important that if confronted with these types of challenging situations that you seek advice and support from your facilitator, mentor or university staff.

Coaching tips

- Inform your educator, mentor or nurse unit manager immediately if you become aware of the presence of someone you know when on a clinical placement.

- Refer to education and healthcare policies and guidelines. Policy directives may mean you are not to have direct responsibility for the care of a patient you know, or you may be requested to complete your clinical placement in an alternative clinical area.

- Keep interactions with patients you know to a minimum.

- Remember always to maintain complete confidentiality regarding the admission and care of all patients, including people you know.

- Review Chapter 2 where the legal concepts of privacy and confidentiality are covered in more detail.

References

Aiken LH, Clarke SP, Cheung RB, et al. Educational levels of hospital nurses and surgical patient mortality. *JAMA*. 2003;290(12):1617-1620.

Alfaro-LeFevre R. *Critical thinking, clinical reasoning and clinical judgement: a practical approach to outcome-focused thinking.* 5th ed. St Louis: Elsevier; 2013.

Baly M. *As Miss Nightingale said…* London: Scutari Press; 1991.

Banning M. Clinical reasoning and its application to nursing: concepts and research studies. *Nurse Educ Pract.* 2008;8:177-183.

Boud D. Avoiding the traps: seeking good practice in the use of self-assessment and reflection in professional courses. *Social Work Education.* 1999;18(2):121-132.

Castillo R, Salguero JM, Fernandez-Berrocal P, et al. Effects of an emotional intelligence intervention on aggression and empathy among adolescents. *J Adolesc.* 2013;36:883-892.

Croskerry P. The importance of cognitive errors in diagnosis and strategies to minimize them. *Academic Medicine.* 2003;78(8):1-6.

Crow GL. Knowing self. In: Bower FL, ed. *Nurses taking the lead: personal qualities of effective leadership.* Philadelphia: WB Saunders; 2000:15-37.

Dahnke M, Dreher M. Defining ethics and applying theories. In: Lachman V, ed. *Applied ethics in nursing.* New York: Springer; 2006.

Driscoll J. *Practising clinical supervision. A reflective approach.* Edinburgh: Ballière Tindall; 2000.

Elkovich K, Barrett P. When whistle blowing seems like the only option. In: Levett-Jones T, ed. *Critical conversations for patient safety: an essential guide for health professionals.* Sydney: Pearson; 2014.

Elstein A, Bordage J. Psychology of clinical reasoning. In: Dowie J, Elstein A, eds. *Professional judgment: a reader in clinical decision-making.* New York: Cambridge University Press; 1991.

Ericsson K, Whyte A, Ward J. Expert performance in nursing: reviewing research on expertise in nursing within the framework of the expert-performance approach. *Adv Nurs Sci.* 2007;30(1):58-71.

Freshwater F. Reflective practice the state of the art. In: Freshwater D, Taylor BJ, Sherwood G, eds. *International textbook of reflective practice in nursing.* Oxford: Blackwell Publishing/Sigma Theta Tau International Honor Society of Nursing; 2008.

Goleman D. *Emotional intelligence.* London: Bloomsbury; 1996.

Goleman D. *Working with emotional intelligence.* London: Bloomsbury; 1998.

Hoffman K. *A comparison of decision-making by 'expert' and 'novice' nurses in the clinical setting, monitoring patient haemodynamic status post abdominal aortic aneurysm surgery.* Unpublished PhD thesis, Sydney: University of Technology; 2007.

Johnstone M. *Bioethics: a nursing perspective.* 5th ed. Sydney: Churchill Livingstone; 2009.

Levett-Jones T. *Belongingness: a pivotal precursor to optimising the learning of nursing students in the clinical environment.* Newcastle: Unpublished PhD Thesis. The University of Newcastle; 2007.

Levett-Jones T, ed. *Clinical Reasoning: learning how to think like a nurse*. Frenchs Forrest: Pearson; 2013.

Levett-Jones T, Hoffman K. Clinical reasoning—what it is and why it matters. In: Levett-Jones T, ed. *Clinical reasoning: learning how to think like a nurse*. Frenchs Forrest: Pearson; 2013.

McCaffery M, Rolling Ferrell B, Paseo C. Nurses' personal opinions about patients' pain and their effect on recorded assessments and titration of opioid doses. *Pain Manag Nurs*. 2000;1(3):79-87.

McCarthy M. Detecting acute confusion in older adults: comparing clinical reasoning of nurses working in acute, long-term, and community health care environments. *Res Nurs Health*. 2003;26:203-212.

Mezirow J. Understanding transformation theory. *AEQ*. 1994;44(4):222-232.

New Zealand Nurses' Organisation. *Code of ethics*. Online. Available: <http://www.nzno.org.nz>; 2010 Accessed 23.02.14.

Nursing Council of New Zealand. *Guidelines: professional boundaries 2012*. Online. Available <http://nursing council.org.nz>; 2012 Accessed 2.09.14.

Nursing and Midwifery Board of Australia (NMBA). *National competency standards for the registered nurse*. Online. Available: <www.nmba.org.au>; 2006 Accessed 23.02.14.

Nursing and Midwifery Board of Australia (NMBA). *Code of ethics for nurses in Australia*. Online. Available: <www.nmba.org.au>; 2008 Accessed 23.02.14.

Nursing and Midwifery Board of Australia (NMBA). *A nurse's guide to professional boundaries*. Online. Available: <www.nmba.org.au>; 2010 Accessed 23.02.14.

O'Grady E, Dempsey L, Fabby C. Anger: a common form of psychological distress among patients at the end of life. *International Journal of Palliative Care*. 2012;18(12):592-596.

Palmer L. Ethical and legal dimensions of clinical reasoning: Caring for a person who is refusing tratement. In: Levett-Jones T, ed. *Clinical reasoning: learning how to think like a nurse*. Frenchs Forrest: Pearson; 2013.

Paul R, Elder L. *The thinker's guide for students on how to study and learn a discipline*. California: Foundation for Critical Thinking Press; 2007.

Peplau HE. *Interpersonal relations in nursing*. New York: Putman; 1952.

Ray S. Whistleblowing and organizational ethics. *Nurs Ethics*. 2006;13(4):438-445.

Rubenfeld M, Scheffer B. *Critical thinking tactics for nurses*. Boston: Jones and Bartlett; 2006.

Scheffer B, Rubenfeld M. A consensus statement on critical thinking in nursing. *J Nurs Educ*. 2000;39: 352-359.

Stone T. *Swearing: impact on nurses and implications for therapeutic practice*. Unpublished PhD thesis. Newcastle: The University of Newcastle; 2009.

Tanner C. Thinking like a nurse: a research-based model of clinical judgement in nursing. *J Nurs Educ*. 2006;45(6):204-211.

van Manen M. *Researching lived experience*. New York: State University of New York Press; 1990.

Varcoe C, Pauly B, Storch J, et al. Nurses' perceptions of morally distressing situations. *Nurs Ethics*. 2012; 19(4):488-500.

Wilson R, Runciman WB, Gibberd RW, et al. The Quality in Australian Health Care Study. *Med J Aust*. 1995;163:458-471.

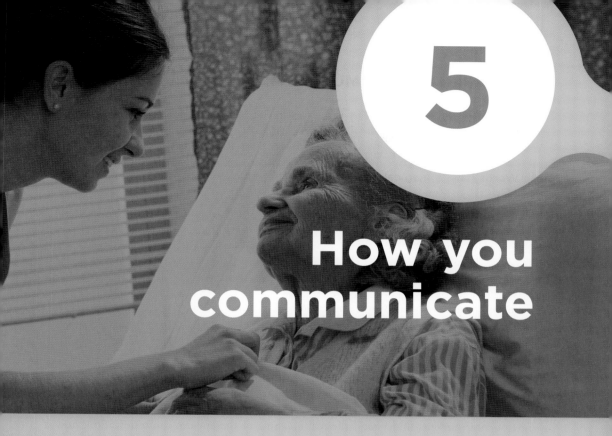

5

How you communicate

What we are missing! What opportunities of understanding we let pass by because at a single decisive moment we were, with all our knowledge, lacking in the simple virtue of a full human presence.

Karl Jasper (cited in Sonneman 1959, p. 375).

INTRODUCTION

In this chapter we add another important layer of knowledge, skills and insights to your repertoire of clinical attributes. We describe how you can make meaningful contributions to patient care through sensitive attention to the way you communicate, both with patients and with members of the healthcare team. The relationship between communication and patient safety is then highlighted and the attributes of therapeutic and interprofessional communication discussed. We also describe the ways in which nurses can define and promote their profession by effectively using their 'nursing voice'. Later in the chapter the use of information and communication technology and the pitfalls and possibilities of using social media are outlined.

THERAPEUTIC COMMUNICATION

SOMETHING TO THINK ABOUT

Words have a magical power. They can bring either the greatest happiness or deepest despair.
Sigmund Freud—founder of psychoanalysis

Communication connects people and creates social bonds, which in turn facilitate survival. A baby learns to cry to elicit a response from their mother when they are hungry or uncomfortable. Over time they develop words to communicate specific needs. Across the lifespan, we communicate not only our basic physical needs and wants but also our most complex, intimate emotional needs.

No doubt you have chosen a career in nursing because you relate well to people and enjoy communicating. You may think you already have excellent 'people skills', and you may wonder why we have included a section on therapeutic communication in our book. Few nursing students understand the real meaning of therapeutic communication, how it differs from social communication and the impact it has on the people for whom they care. Few realise that effective communication can actually be a form of therapy and a key factor in patient safety. Effective communication impacts on patient outcomes in many ways. Studies have demonstrated a relationship between therapeutic communication and, for example: chronic disease management (Rungby & Brock 2010); compliance with medication and rehabilitation programs (Rossiter et al. 2014); a reduction in stress and anxiety; pain management; and self-management (Harms 2007). However, as with all forms of therapy, therapeutic communication requires knowledge, a defined skill set and practice (lots of practice!).

How is therapeutic communication different from how you communicate in your everyday life? Therapeutic communication occurs when the nurse effectively uses communication techniques and processes with a patient in a goal-directed way. Therapeutic communication is person-centred, focusing on the patient's needs not the nurse's; it is not a mutual sharing of feelings or thoughts. When therapeutic communication is utilised the nurse responds not only to the content of the patient's message but also to the feelings expressed through verbal and non-verbal communication. Therapeutic communication requires active listening, attending to the patient, hearing what is being said and what is not being said, and communicating back to the patient in a way that indicates the nurse has heard and understood the message. This type of communication requires emotional intelligence (see Chapter 4), energy and concentration. It conveys an attitude of genuine caring and concern. Therapeutic communication requires you to develop a broad range of skills and techniques such as:

- prompting
- instructing
- probing using open-ended and closed questions

- expressing empathy
- the use of silence
- non-verbal behaviours such as touch
- paraphrasing or restating
- seeking clarification
- providing information
- encouraging and acknowledging
- confronting
- respect for personal space
- focusing
- reflecting
- summarising (Day et al. 2015).

For nurses to provide effective care and ensure patient safety, it is imperative that the capacity for therapeutic communication is enhanced by suspending personal judgements and biases and authentically demonstrating respect and empathy for the person requiring care (Rossiter et al. 2014). We need to ask the question: How do we as nurses 'be with' our patients in a way that enhances the therapeutic relationship and that invokes trust and confidence? Remember, if your patient doesn't feel safe with you or doesn't trust you, they will not tell you everything; likewise, they may not follow through on your instructions for treatment (Rossiter et al. 2014). Refer to Box 5.1 for a list of attributes of a therapeutic relationship.

| **Box 5.1** | Attributes of a therapeutic relationship |

A therapeutic relationship:

- is a partnership between a patient and a nurse, focused on the patient's healthcare needs or goals
- considers people to be autonomous individuals capable of decision making
- considers the person's culture, values, beliefs and spiritual needs
- respects patient confidentiality
- focuses on the promotion of self-management and independence
- is based on trust, respect and acceptance.

Source: Day et al. 2015

SOMETHING TO THINK ABOUT

The greatest problem with communication is the illusion that it has been accomplished.
George Bernard Shaw—Irish playwright

Therapeutic communication does not just happen. As with all forms of therapy it is a skill that takes time to learn and deliberate practice to master. However, the benefits for your patient are worth the investment.

While a full explanation of therapeutic communication is beyond the remit of this book, you will undoubtedly have opportunities to learn more about this essential nursing skill at university and you will have many opportunities to practise it when undertaking placements. You should also refer to the Nursing and Midwifery Board of Australia (NMBA) *National competency standards for the registered nurse* (2006), Collaborative and Therapeutic Practice Domain, where the expectations of the nursing profession in relation to communication are clearly explained.

We also recommend you access the following resources to enhance your understanding of the attributes and importance of therapeutic communication:

- Day J, Levett-Jones T, Kenny R. Communicating. In: Berman A, Synder S, Levett-Jones T, et al., eds. *Kozier and Erb's fundamentals of nursing*. Sydney: Pearson; 2015.

- Levett-Jones T. *Critical conversations for patient safety: an essential guide for health professionals*. Sydney: Pearson; 2014.

SOMETHING TO THINK ABOUT

Improving patient endurance with comfort talk

Seriously injured patients undergoing life-saving procedures after trauma often experience pain and fear that is overwhelming. They vocalise their distress, withdraw from painful activities and may be combative towards members of the healthcare team. In this context, the goal of care is to stabilise the patient, minimise the effect of injuries and maximise survival. Comfort behaviours used by nurses are described by patients as their lifeline. 'Comfort talk' combined with the nurse's posture, touch and gaze enable patient to endure extraordinary pain associated with trauma care. 'Comfort talk' keeps patients focused on the minute-by-minute progression of the care ('Nearly finished ... then we're done'). It enables patients to prepare for the next procedure and orients them by providing information about their condition and the necessity for care ('You've got a very bad cut here ... we'll have to clean and suture it'). Critical care is able to be given quickly and safely by assisting the patient to remain in control and endure by using comfort talk.

Source: Morse & Proctor 1998

INTERPROFESSIONAL AND INTRAPROFESSIONAL COMMUNICATION

Every aspect of patient care depends upon how well health professionals communicate with each other and the patients they care for. A groundbreaking study undertaken over a decade ago identified that more than 70% of adverse patient outcomes were caused by communication errors (Joint Commission 2004). It is estimated that this figure is even higher in the complex world of contemporary healthcare (Lapkin et al., in press).

Interprofessional communication is focused on preventing adverse events and promoting patient wellbeing. Patient-safe communication is the way that competent health professionals work collaboratively to collect and share information and to clarify and verify accurate interpretations of patient information (Levett-Jones et al. 2014). Effective interprofessional communication (between health professionals from different disciplines) and intraprofessional communication (between health professionals from the same discipline) are increasingly recognised as core competencies for all health professionals. Unsafe communication is considered to be a breach of professional standards and a leading cause of litigation (Trede et al. 2012).

It is important to realise that the hierarchical nature of healthcare environments too often works against effective interprofessional and intraprofessional communication (see box below). Power differentials and traditional healthcare cultures can make it difficult for health professionals to be assertive and raise concerns when they are worried about patients (Levett-Jones et al. 2014). However, confident and well-educated health professionals can use clearly agreed upon communication processes that help improve communication and avoid the tendency to speak indirectly or disrespectfully.

SOMETHING TO THINK ABOUT

Sometimes you're fumbling your way through and you look to the nurses for a bit of a clue of what to do. I had a situation when there was a patient who I couldn't get a cannula into. He was dehydrated, but he was taking in fluids, and his diarrhoea had stopped. I tried a couple of times, went away and came back, and then decided we were just going to go with oral fluids. And the nurse sort of made this face, but she didn't say anything. I said to her, 'You don't look very happy with that. What do you think? What's the problem?' And so she sort of exploded then and said she thought it was really a bad idea and that 'we really have to get a line into this patient' and that he was 'going to go downhill if we don't'. So after she said that it sort of felt like quite an easy decision ... I been sitting on the fence and didn't really know what to do. But I wished that she'd said something, and not just sat there and made a face, because if I hadn't seen it, what would have happened to that patient?

Source: Levett-Jones et al. 2014

SOMETHING TO THINK ABOUT

Read the excerpt below and the linked digital story. Then reflect on how effective interprofessional and intraprofessional communication would have made a difference to how the events unfolded. Consider what you would have done if you were one of the nurses involved in Vanessa's story and what you will do in clinical practice as a result of what you have learnt about communication.

In 1989 a 16-year-old girl died in a large metropolitan teaching hospital in Sydney. Her death resulted from a series of system and human errors. However, had the health professionals involved in Vanessa's care communicated in an effective way her death would not have resulted. Magistrate Milovanovich, the deputy state coroner of New South Wales, made the following statement in relation to the findings of the coronial inquest following Vanessa's death:

The death of Vanessa Anderson at the very young age of 16 years was a tragic and avoidable death ... the circumstances of Vanessa's death should constantly remain in the forefront of the minds of all medical practitioners, nursing staff and hospital administrators. Vanessa's case should be used as a precedent to highlight how individual errors of judgment, failure to communicate, failure to record accurately and poor management of staff resources, cumulatively led to the worst possible outcome for Vanessa and her family.

Inquest into the death of Vanessa Anderson, Coroner's Court, Westmead, Sydney, Australia, 24 January 2004

Go to the following website to see a re-enactment of Vanessa Anderson's story: <www.ipeforqum.com.au/modules>.

COMMUNICATING AS A PROFESSIONAL NURSE

SOMETHING TO THINK ABOUT

Envision how things would be if the voice and visibility of nursing were commensurate with the size and importance of the nursing profession care.

Buresh & Gordon 2013, p. 13

The public holds nurses in very high regard. Opinion polls indicate that nursing is one of the most highly rated professions in terms of honesty and ethics (Swift 2013). However, when people think of registered nurses they are more inclined to dwell on their kindness and caring than on their knowledge, expertise or professionalism. The public's image of the nursing profession is linked to nurses' ability to articulate their experience, skills and expertise:

> Let your eagerness, enthusiasm and commitment to nursing be reflected in your voice and body language. When nurses speak with passion and conviction—rather than in cautious and passive tones—they convince the public that nurses are important professionals who cannot easily be replaced.
>
> Buresh & Gordon 2013, p. 120

Introducing yourself to other health professionals

Nurses have a choice about the way they present themselves to patients, families, doctors, other clinicians and the general public. They can present themselves in ways that assert their personal and professional identity, or they can remain part of the wider, undifferentiated healthcare services industry. They can highlight their clinical competence or they can conceal it. Each day in the workplace, what nurses say and do will either elicit the respect and collegial treatment their professional standing deserves, or undermine it.

While caring for patients and families, or interacting with other members of the healthcare team, nurses convey messages about their own respect for the status of nursing. Some of these messages are explicit; others are more implicit, delivered through presentation, body language, tone of voice and conversational style. For example, if a nurse thinks it advisable to consult a doctor, she or he can inform the patient by saying, 'I'll discuss this with the doctor'. By using these words nurses imply that they have clinical knowledge and judgement, and see themselves as doctors' colleagues. Alternatively, nurses can communicate in a more subservient way by saying, 'I'll have to ask the doctor'.

When contacting a doctor, a nurse can establish collegiality by beginning the conversation with the words 'Hello, Dr Smith, this is Sarah O'Shea, Mrs Johnson's nurse. She is experiencing chest pain and I think …' Alternatively, she can apologise for the interruption and cast herself in an inferior role by beginning 'I'm so sorry to bother you Dr Smith, but this is Sarah, Mrs Johnson's nurse …'. The way that health professionals communicate with each other during these type of interactions has been shown to have a direct impact on patient safety. Communication tools such as ISBAR (Identify, Situation, Background, Assessment, Recommendations) have been implemented to provide a clear structure and to improve health professionals' confidence and assertiveness when communicating with other staff members (see Box 5.2).

Introducing yourself to patients and families

The way nurses introduce themselves to patients and their families can have a significant impact on how they are perceived. You can introduce yourself with a firm handshake, provide your full name, tell them you are a nursing student from the University of …. and explain your role in the patient's care. Or you can simply say, 'Hello, I'm John, and I'm caring for you today' and leave it at that.

Most patients meeting you for the first time have few visual cues about your identity and role. Your introduction is your best opportunity to let people know you are a nursing student with clinical skills and knowledge (Buresh & Gordon 2013).

Box 5.2	ISBAR

Safe healthcare delivery depends on effective communication between health professionals. There will be times when you need to relay your concerns about a patient's deteriorating clinical condition to senior staff. These are not times for vague requests and inadequate or incorrect information. You need to become confident and skilled in communicating with members of the healthcare team so you can signal your need for immediate action and support when required. Use of acronyms such as ISBAR have been reported to be effective in streamlining the way health professionals communicate during telephone calls and patient handover and in increasing patient safety. Acronyms provide a framework for communicating in a consistent way and are particularly useful for beginning nurses.

I	Identify	Self—name, position, location Patient—name, age, gender	'This is … from … ward.' 'I'm calling about Mr Levi …'
S	Situation	Explain what has happened to trigger this conversation	'The reason I'm calling is …' If urgent, say so: 'This is urgent; the patient's O_2 saturation levels are 90% and systolic BP 90.'
B	Background	Admission date, diagnosis, relevant history, investigations, what has been done so far	'He is day 2 post-op after colorectal resection …'
A	Assessment	Give a summary of the patient's condition or situation. Explain what you think the problem is (if you can)	'I'm not sure what the problem is, but the patient is deteriorating. His vital signs are …'
R	Request and/or recommendation	State your request	'I need help urgently. Can you come now?'

Source: Iedema 2014

First name basis?

In some clinical contexts it has become common for nurses to use only their first names when introducing themselves to patients, visitors or doctors, and some name badges bear only first names. Although the use of first names may vary depending on the context of practice and the policies of the institution, can you imagine doctors introducing themselves by their first names only? Why, then, is there an imbalance between these two professions? If nurses continue to uphold and reinforce these identification practices, it suggests that nurses regard doctors as superior in the healthcare environment. We know this is not the real intention of nurses who use only their first names. Mostly, they are doing it to develop a friendly and informal relationship with their patients, and to show them they are 'on their side' or 'an equal'. Unfortunately, this often misconstrues what patients really want and need from a nurse. They do not want you to be their friend; they want a nurse with knowledge and skills.

> Your introduction is your best opportunity to let people know that you are a nurse—a serious professional with important clinical knowledge. Being serious and professional is not synonymous with being distant and aloof. It simply means presenting yourself as a knowledgeable, expert caregiver. This presentation tends to reassure patients rather than alienate them.
>
> (Buresh & Gordon 2013, p. 87)

For some nurses, it is not unusual to address their patients, particularly if they are elderly, using endearments such as sweetie, pet, darling, angel or lovey (Gardner et al. 2001). However, this is not person-centred language and many people will be offended by being addressed in this manner, so don't assume it is acceptable. A good rule is to simply ask a patient if he would prefer you to use his given name (e.g. John) or address him more formally (Mr Smith).

DIVERSITY AND ITS IMPACT ON CLINICAL COMMUNICATION

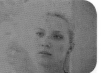

STUDENT STORY
'I think language is the most important thing'
Felisa's story (Felisa is from China)

Being an international student I'm supposed to learn the language to be able to communicate with other people like in handover or when I give out medications … I need language. If I have a question, if I need to read … I need language. It is very, very important. I think language is the first of the first, the most important thing.

Source: Dickson 2013, p. 96

This section is related to the topic of cultural competence discussed in Chapter 3. It is written especially for international students who will need to negotiate the complexities of clinical practice in an unfamiliar country. However, it will also be beneficial to all students because we will all work with people from a range of cultural backgrounds at some point. We hope this brief overview complements what you learn in class about the diversity of contemporary practice settings and helps you become accustomed to the many cultural factors that can influence your clinical experience. Without this knowledge, miscommunication is common and learning possibilities are sometimes reduced.

The nursing workforce has also become increasingly diverse over the past decade. Workforce shortages have led to recruitment of nurses from many countries, and in 2011 the number of nurses born overseas was 33% (Australian Bureau of Statistics 2013). Additionally, the percentage of international students in Australian universities is the highest of any OECD country (OECD 2010); in some nursing programs more than 20% of students are from overseas. No longer are nursing students a homogenous white female group; instead, contemporary nursing programs are composed of heterogeneous male and female students from a multitude of cultural backgrounds (Dickson 2013).

The increasing numbers of international students in academic programs such as nursing have had a positive impact on our ability to appreciate and understand different cultures. The diversity and richness that international students and nurses bring to the academic and clinical environment enhances the learning opportunities of all students and staff. However, while most students may, at some stage, experience difficulties related to their clinical placement, these may be exacerbated by language and cultural differences. If this happens it is important to reflect and try to analyse the root cause of the problem so that appropriate support, guidance and teaching can be provided. Reflect on the stories below and examine the issues of concern. The coaching tips provide practical guidance and advice.

Receptive communication

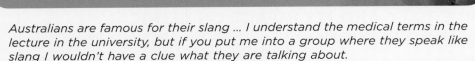

STUDENT STORY
'I wouldn't have a clue what they are talking about'
Milky's story (Milky is from China)

Australians are famous for their slang … I understand the medical terms in the lecture in the university, but if you put me into a group where they speak like slang I wouldn't have a clue what they are talking about.

Source: Dickson 2013, p. 100

Do you sometimes find it hard to understand what your patients or nursing colleagues are saying to you? Local accents, shortened, fast speech and the use of colloquialisms can cause significant difficulties for nurses and students from a non-English speaking background. Misunderstandings between you and others may occur if you do not readily acknowledge when you have not understood or have only partially understood a conversation. Most importantly, patient safety may be jeopardised if you are not perfectly clear about what is being asked of you. Initially, it may be culturally difficult for you to do this, but keep in mind that in Australia and New Zealand it is not considered disrespectful to question an individual in authority or to ask someone to repeat what they have said. Nor is it considered a 'failure' on your part if you have not understood something. On the contrary, clinicians will expect you to ask questions and to ask for clarification whenever you need to.

STUDENT STORY
'Sometimes it is so hard to understand'
Manoj's story (Manoj is from India)

Most of the patients are from English-speaking countries but there are some from other parts of the world such as Poland, The Netherlands, Greece … and their way of speaking is all together different. The Greeks speak English with a different accent and the Polish speak English with a different accent. Sometimes it is so hard to understand.

Source: Dickson 2103, p. 110

- If you want to confirm your understanding of an instruction or discussion, try paraphrasing—for example, 'Can I confirm that you'd like me to take Mrs Smith to the shower on a commode because of her low blood pressure?'

- Ask someone to explain any colloquial terms you do not understand (fellow students are usually willing to do this).

- If you are unsure of healthcare terminology related to your patients ask questions and be prepared to do some research.

- Remember, nodding or silence following a conversation may be taken to indicate that you fully understood what was being said, even if the reverse is true.

Expressive communication

STUDENT STORY

'Sometimes you want to say something but it just doesn't come out'
Yvonne's story (Yvonne is from Nepal)

Coming from a different background sometimes I can't even speak properly ... at times I just get numb. Because English is not my first language I have to think before I speak; it makes things difficult and awkward. Sometimes you want to say something but it just doesn't come out.

Source: Dickson 2013, p. 98

- Observing nursing staff communicating effectively with one another and with patients will allow you to clarify expectations and build upon what you already know.

- Thoughtfully reflect on the nurse–patient interactions you observe. Consider what made the interactions effective (or ineffective). How and why was humour used? What colloquialisms and terms need clarification?

- Make the most of opportunities to practise communicating with patients and staff.

- Do not hesitate to ask your clinical educator or mentor to provide detailed feedback on your communication skills.

- Most educational institutions have student support services that provide English language tuition. Avail yourself of this opportunity if you require additional help. Alternatively, seek English language tuition from external providers such as community colleges.

Do you sometimes find it difficult or frustrating trying to make yourself understood by patients or nursing colleagues? During your studies you will be expected to become increasingly fluent in the English language, familiar with colloquialisms and conversant with the professional language used to communicate with health professionals but still have the ability to switch to less formal language when needed—for example, when conversing with patients.

Written communication

Is it sometimes difficult to understand what you read or to find the English words for what you want to write? Both international and local students can experience difficulties with reading and writing. Patients' notes, referral letters, medication charts and other forms of professional documentation may be especially problematic as students learn to use appropriate language and grammar.

Coaching tips

- Develop a glossary of terms and their definitions (professional terminology as well as more conversational terms); add to it regularly, and use it often.
- Practise, practise, practise! Try writing a nursing report on notepaper and asking someone you respect and trust to critique it for you before you write in a patient's notes.
- Reading nursing journals will help you to develop your fluency in English and your professional vocabulary, and will build on what you already know.
- Reading good-quality English-language novels set in Australia or New Zealand will improve your literacy and grammar, and help you to better understand colloquialisms and local culture. Ask your librarian to recommend appropriate novels.
- Remember that in nursing reports you must always sign your name in English.

Cultural and professional issues

Are you finding the clinical culture in Australia or New Zealand confusing and stressful? If you have no previous experience with these healthcare systems it may be difficult at first to understand the complexity of the structures and values that operate within the organisation. The interactions between you and patients or other health professionals may present unique issues. This not only applies to international students but also to local students who care for patients from culturally and linguistically diverse cultures. Misunderstandings may involve religion, gender and age-related issues, as well as language. Sometimes a lack of understanding and tolerance on the part of some clinical staff and fellow students may have a negative impact on the ability of international students to fit into and feel accepted in the clinical environment. Additionally, the roles, and responsibilities undertaken by registered nurses in Australia or New Zealand may be very different from what you are used to, and you may find this disconcerting (see Cheska's story).

STUDENT STORY

'If you are a nurse you are going to be proud to say I'm a nurse'
Cheska's story (Cheska is from the Philippines)

There is a big difference between nursing in Australia and the Philippines. [In the Philippines] they are not really professionals; they are just like assistants to the doctor. They don't have their own professional identity. But here in Australia if you are a nurse you are going to be proud to say I'm a nurse.

Source: Dickson 2013, p. 121

Coaching tips

- Many educational institutions have dedicated courses, or an orientation program, to prepare international students for the cultural differences they may encounter. Local community colleges also provide programs to assist with reading, writing and speaking. Make the most of these learning opportunities as well as the opportunities to interact with local students.

- Join local sporting, musical or recreational clubs to increase your opportunities for socialising with people from different backgrounds.

- During your clinical placement experiences it is important that you express any concerns you have, even though it may be difficult to do so. Sharing your worries with someone you trust will mean you can be supported and guided. Sadly, not all students, staff or patients will be sensitive to different health beliefs, customs and cultural and religious practices. If you experience discrimination, subtle or obvious, you need to discuss it with your educator or academic staff member. All Australian educational and healthcare institutions have policies regarding discrimination and people who can advocate for you. Your concerns will be taken seriously.

- Seek out a peer mentor to work with during your studies. This should be a person who can support your development in the English language. Spend time together focusing on language development and understanding.

- All students (those from Australia, New Zealand and other countries) should practise in a culturally competent way (review *Cultural competence* in Chapter 3). However, the attitudes that underpin cultural competence should also influence how you behave at university and in your everyday life.

- *Everyday English for nursing* (Grice 2003) is an excellent resource to help you develop your English language skills and Hally (2009) has also written an informative guide for international nursing students studying in Australia and New Zealand.

USING PROFESSIONAL LANGUAGE

Nurses must be able to describe the care they give and the clinical decisions they make (Buresh & Gordon 2013). In discussions with colleagues, patients, their significant others and the public, the language that nurses use reflects on their professional standing. Nursing students are recognised as a part of a group of health professionals and are expected to behave according to the conventions of the nursing profession.

Throughout your career you will accumulate a lot of professional and jargon-based words and statements that will become a normal part of your practice language. Nursing jargon refers to words that are used by nurses when they talk about their practice. These words may exclude people who are unfamiliar with their use, so choose your words carefully when you speak to people who do not have a nursing background. Distinguish between what you say to health workers and what you say to a layperson. Colloquial language, or slang, is often referred to as conversational speech without constraint. While appropriate in some contexts, its use should be minimised in the practice environment.

As you progress through your nursing program, you will develop a wide repertoire of professional terminology. Give careful consideration to your audience to ensure you use the most appropriate language in each situation. The inappropriate use of nursing terminology will completely change the meaning of your message. Abbreviations must be approved by the institution in which you are undertaking your placement. Some words that are commonly abbreviated can have very different meanings within various contexts of practice (e.g. 'SB' may be an abbreviation for 'seen by' or 'short of breath'). Clinical errors can occur as a result of this type of miscommunication.

Coaching tips

- Reflect upon language used in professional situations and how it affects others.
- Reflect on the language you use: words, selected statements (informal and formal), tone and volume.
- Consider who you are speaking to and their background, age, culture, medical condition, status and knowledge.
- Consider whether the language you use is person-centred.
- Think about whether your words and language are appropriate in each situation.
- Select words and terms that cannot easily be misinterpreted.
- Give people time to consider your words and to respond to your questions.
- Explain medical and nursing terms to patients using language that is easily understood.
- Be aware that the way a word is interpreted may be influenced by the thoughts, feelings and beliefs people may have about that word (e.g. drug versus medication).
- Avoid the use of colloquial and coarse language in the practice environment. (Many people are offended by swearing and use of religious terms such as 'oh my god'.)

Coaching tips (cont'd)

- Consider the effect of your words on others (some words may convey a false sense of urgency to a patient).
- Learn the meaning of medical terminology and use the terms accurately (e.g. words ending in -ectomy, -ology, -oscopy and -otomy).
- Make a list of accepted abbreviations. Access and become familiar with the Australian Commission of Safety and Quality in Health Care's recommendations for *Terminology, abbreviations and symbols used in the prescribing and administration of medications* at <http://www.safetyandquality.gov.au/wp-content/uploads/2012/01/32060v2.pdf>.
- Listen and learn from the way your role model uses professional language.

Your voice in the clinical environment

Your voice is one of your most effective communication tools. You should be aware how you use this tool, and make it an efficient component in your repertoire of skills. Reflect upon the pitch and tone of your voice so that you are aware of how you come across to others. The following are some examples of inappropriate use of one's voice:

- a nurse calling down the corridor
- speaking so quietly that your patients cannot hear what you are saying
- a group of nurses laughing loudly at the nurses' station.

Clinical environments are different in structure and design. They can be small, intimate rooms where patients are interviewed, or rooms attached to a long corridor. Corridors echo and the sound of people's voices can carry over long distances and traverse hard surfaces such as doors and walls. A comment made to a patient in one room may be very appropriate, but if the comment is overheard in an adjoining room it may unnecessarily frighten or distress someone. Think carefully about the pitch of your voice when talking to others.

Pitch of voice is critical to the development of appropriate communication skills. A loud voice is easily heard but also easily overheard. Some people find that their voice projects well and other people have no trouble hearing what they say. People with this type of voice need to be mindful of how far their voice carries. If you are aware that you have a loud voice, try standing next to the person you are talking to rather than speaking from a distance. This technique has the effect of reducing the projection factor you add to your voice when speaking at a distance (even short distances). Use eye contact to help direct your voice.

However, a soft voice can be difficult to hear and detracts from the message being conveyed. It can be a source of frustration for the listener. If you have a very soft voice, remember that any physical barriers (e.g. masks or curtains around a bed) may render your voice difficult to hear. Keep what you say clear, simple and straightforward. Connect with those to whom you are speaking to engage their attention (maintain eye contact, position yourself, use appropriate gestures). Practise voice projection to enable your voice to be heard within a group. Move forward in a group to engage people in the conversation so that you are speaking within a closer range.

Accents have a powerful effect on the listener's ability to understand what is being said. If you speak with an accent, you may need to slow down your speech to allow the listener to 'attune' to the accent initially so that communication is effective.

- Assess your voice—is it too loud or too soft for effective communication? Try recording yourself and then listening to how you sound. Also, ask family or friends to give you some feedback about how you sound.
- Walk up to people to communicate rather than speaking loudly.
- Consider the number of people who need to hear you and the type of information that is important to convey. Reflect upon the situation and modify your voice to suit.
- Be aware of how you sound during spoken communication practices. Is your voice squeaky, high-pitched, growling or guttural?
- Consider how fast or slowly you speak, and the associated pitch of your voice.
- Be careful of how your voice projects in long corridors or large rooms.
- If you are concerned about your voice and the impact it has on others, seek feedback and try to improve your speech by attending training sessions or public speaking groups.

DOCUMENTATION AND LEGAL ISSUES

Quality documentation is essential to patient safety; it is a way of recording the care given to patients and ensuring communication between members of the healthcare team is effective. Accurate and timely documentation is a requirement of all health professionals. Documentation may make or break the defence of a hospital and staff if legal action is instigated following a critical incident or unexplained death. Currently, Australia has one of the highest incidences of medical litigation in the developed world. Some points you should consider:

- Documentation is considered to be the most important evidence in a potential legal action, and therefore its significance should not be underestimated.
- Legal action may be initiated many years after a critical incident occurs. Memories of witnesses will obviously fade, and therefore accurate documentation may be crucial to the outcome of the case.
- Accurate documentation ensures that your nursing report demonstrates evidence of the care given to your patients, as well as providing a means of communication between health professionals.
- Accurate documentation means more relevant documentation, not more extensive documentation.
- Quality documentation saves you time and may protect you from potential litigation.
- The best answer to litigation is concise, accurate, objective and contemporaneous documentation.

- Reports should be concise. Avoid verbosity and 'double charting'. Most healthcare organisations have a policy that specifies that only deviations from normal are documented in the patient progress notes.

- Avoid unnecessarily long words and sentences. Use care plans and clinical pathways as adjuncts to progress notes, but do not duplicate information.

- Reports should be accurate. You should distinguish between what you personally observe and what is related to you by another person (hearsay)—for example, 'The patient stated that she had slipped over', not 'The patient slipped over'. Unless you have actually witnessed the incident, the patient's complaint is hearsay and must be reported as such.

- Reports should be objective. Avoid using the word 'appears'. You should record what you actually see, not what you think you see—for example, 'The patient appears to be in shock' should instead be documented as 'The patient is pale and sweating, hypotensive, BP 80/40, tachycardic, pulse 140, with peripheral cyanosis' or 'The patient was observed at two-hourly intervals during the night, and when observed was sleeping', not 'Patient appears to have slept all night'.

- Documentation should be contemporaneous. It should be written as close as possible to the time when the incident or treatment occurred. Memories fade, and often one incident is followed closely by a series of incidents, particularly if a patient's condition deteriorates and a number of treatments are initiated. Trying to put this in sequence at the end of the shift can be confusing and lead to inaccuracies.

- Always sign, print your name and include your designation at the end of your report. Most healthcare facilities require that a student's documentation is countersigned by a registered nurse.

- Documentation should be specific. Say exactly what you mean—for example, 'Patient experienced a sudden onset of severe breathlessness following ambulation, respiratory rate 34, oxygen saturations 90%', not 'Patient feeling breathless'.

- Written documentation should be legible, with correct spelling and grammar. Nurses often complain about doctors' handwriting, but they, too, may be at fault. If a negligence case is taken to court, your nursing notes may be used as evidence. Imagine how you'd feel if your notes could not be interpreted because of poor legibility. Furthermore, reports filled with misspelt words and incorrect grammar create the same negative impression as illegible handwriting.

Coaching tips (cont'd)

- Document all relevant information. Document any change in the patient's condition, what you observed to support this observation, your follow-up actions and who you notified of the change. Also document if there has been no change in the patient's condition during your shift. Do not document normal observations that have been charted elsewhere, such as vital signs, postoperative observations, voiding or drain patency, but do document if there are any aberrations from normal and what your actions were. The use of clinical pathways and care plans has significantly reduced the need for extensive documentation in progress notes.

- Only accepted abbreviations are to be used. Students work in many different institutions during their clinical placements and later employment. A diversity of abbreviations can lead to confusing and misleading interpretations—for example, the abbreviation 'IUD' can be taken to mean 'intrauterine device' or 'intrauterine death'. Make sure you understand the meaning of any medical and nursing abbreviations used, and include only accepted and easy-to-understand abbreviations in your notes.

- An error should be dealt with by drawing a line through the incorrect entry and initialling it. Total obliteration may suggest that you have something to hide. For the same reason, white-out should not be used.

- Do not make an entry in a patient's notes before checking the name and medical record number (MRN) on the patient's chart. Don't rely on room numbers only. Patients are often moved from room to room and have also been known to 'get into the wrong bed'.

- All omissions should be documented. If you do not carry out an ordered treatment or procedure, always document why it was omitted and who you notified. If nothing is written, it may be presumed that the procedure was simply overlooked. For example, if a patient's hypertensive medication was not administered because the patient's BP was too low, this must be documented in the patient's notes and on the medication chart. The follow-up action and the person notified should be included.

- When you are busy with patient care, documentation may seem to be of secondary importance. However, from a coroner's point of view an incomplete chart may suggest incomplete nursing care. This is not always true, but it is an easy inference to make. You may have performed a nursing procedure and simply forgotten to chart it, but if a dispute arises many years later you will have nothing to back up your version of the facts, assuming you can even remember what you did at the time.

- Be aware that the assumption is made that if something is not documented then it has not been done.

Coaching tips (cont'd)

- Do not make an entry in a patient's notes on behalf of another person.
- Be aware that nurses are practising in an era of consumerism. This has created a more litigious and complaint-oriented society. In order to protect themselves from potential litigation, nurses need high-quality and more relevant documentation. You should always bear in mind that you will be held accountable for the care provided to patients and may be called upon to explain your actions in relation to patient care. Good-quality documentation is part of your accountability and may be the only assistance you can rely upon if asked to explain your professional actions.

PATIENT HANDOVER

SOMETHING TO THINK ABOUT

The quality of a clinical handover directly influences patient safety in the shift that follows.

Source: Garling 2008

The patient handover report (change of shift report) is a communication practice used by nurses and other health professionals to communicate a patient's care requirements, condition and progress at change of shift. A common definition of handover is 'the transfer of professional responsibility and accountability for some or all aspects of care for a patient, or group of patients, to another person or professional group on a temporary or permanent basis' (Australian Medical Association 2007, p S108). The purpose of a patient handover report is to provide continuity of care among nurses who are caring for a patient. They may be given in a verbal, recorded, written or electronic format.

In some institutions handover may be undertaken as patient rounds, with patients and their families also contributing to decision making and care planning. In others, handover may be held in the staffroom or conference room, with nurses from the previous shift joined by nurses for the next shift. In these situations the handover time is an opportunity for nurses to come together to discuss patient care as a team. Because of time constraints, reports are sometimes pre-recorded. The advantage of recording is that nurses can provide their handover at a convenient time during the shift. The disadvantage is that this doesn't allow nurses to clarify and review care as they would in a face-to-face handover.

The handover report shares information about patients and describes the health status of patients, any aberrations from normal, interventions implemented and the effectiveness of interventions (such as analgesia). Information needs to be accurate, objective, concise, logical and to the point.

Handover processes are highly variable and often unreliable, causing clinical handover to be a high-risk area for patient safety (see Box 5.3). Breakdown in the transfer of information or in communication at handover has been identified as one of the most important contributing factors in serious adverse events and is a major preventable cause of patient harm (Iedema 2014). For this reason nursing students need to make the most of opportunities to be present at patient handover and to learn as much as possible about the correct processes. You should also practise giving and receiving handover about your patient's condition and care requirements. Ask your mentor for advice and feedback about your handover.

Box 5.3	High-risk scenarios in clinical handover

A systematic review by Wong et al. (2008) identified some of the high-risk patient handover processes that can result in discontinuity of care, adverse patient outcomes and legal claims of malpractice.

- **Interprofessional handover:** between operating theatre and post-anaesthesia care (recovery) staff and between ambulance and emergency department staff.
- **Inter-departmental handover:** between emergency department and intensive-care staff and emergency department and ward staff (especially where interdepartmental boundaries and/or responsibilities are unclear).
- **Shift-to-shift handover:** risks related to the lack of a clear structure, policy or procedures for handover; interruptions and information overload caused by overly long and detailed handovers.
- **Hospital-to-community and hospital-to-residential care handover:** risks related to poor hospital-to-community discharge processes and incomplete or inaccurate communication resulting in clinical errors and re-hospitalisations.
- **Providing verbal handover only:** depending on memory, can cause a loss of or inaccurate information transfer.
- **The use of non-standard abbreviations:** can cause misunderstandings between health professionals.
- **Patient's characteristics:** complex patient problems receive poorer quality handover than more defined patient conditions.

Coaching tips

- Be on time for shift handover and remain for the entire process.
- Take notes and ask questions about anything you are unsure of.
- Ensure handover notes remain confidential at all times and dispose of the notes correctly before you leave the clinical setting.
- Use a standard format to present your handover report.
- Be respectful of the people you are discussing. Avoid the use of judgemental language, and do not label or stereotype your patients or make negative comments about them.

Coaching tips (cont'd)

- Use correct terminology and abbreviations, professional language and only easily understood and recognised abbreviations.
- Avoid repetition and irrelevant data.
- Discuss with your clinical educator or mentor any issues that need clarification immediately following the report.
- Compare and contrast the different handover techniques you encounter during clinical placement.

ELECTRONIC DOCUMENTATION IN HEALTHCARE

Research suggests that the quality of patient documentation can be enhanced by the introduction of electronic medical records (Australian Commission on Safety and Quality in Health Care 2013). Electronic documentation can help overcome some of the problems associated with a lack of integrated systems and disparate forms and processes. These inconsistencies make it difficult to manage patient journeys effectively during a continuum of care. Poor communication affects all clients, but older people and those with chronic diseases have been identified as particularly vulnerable to the effects of incomplete and inaccurate documentation during admission, discharge, transfer and referral to service providers in the community. This is one of the driving forces behind the transition to electronic documentation.

Too often handwritten documents are 'illegible, incomplete and poorly organised, making it difficult to ensure quality of care' (Tsai & Bond 2008). For example, studies comparing electronic records with paper records in mental health centres reported that electronic records were 40% more complete and 20% faster to retrieve (Tsai & Bond 2008). As a student working in contemporary practice environments, such as community care, aged care and acute care, you will be required to become increasingly confident and competent in using electronic medical records, point-of-care documentation systems, online pathology results and electronic medication administration records (and maintaining the security of this data). *A healthier future for all Australians* (National Health and Hospitals Reform Commission 2009) advocates that quality, safety and efficiency of healthcare is linked to the smart use of data information and that it is imperative that clinicians and healthcare providers are supported to 'get out of paper' and adopt electronic information storage, exchange and decision-support software. These contemporary issues require you to have a sophisticated level of information and communication technology (ICT) skills. This requirement, and some of the issues that impact on ICT competence, are discussed more fully in the next section.

INFORMATION AND COMMUNICATION TECHNOLOGY IN HEALTHCARE AND IN EDUCATION

ICT has the capacity to enable rapid and efficient communication of information across distances to support clinical and educational processes (Jones et al. 2014). The term 'ICT competence' refers to the ability to function with information systems, networks, software and web applications through the use of computers, smart devices and other technologies. In contemporary clinical practice environments ICT skills are advantageous, not only to nurses but also to the patients for whom we care. There is good evidence that ICT skills, appropriately utilised, can have a significant impact on patient outcomes. A requisite level of ICT competence allows nurses to not only access diagnostic information (e.g. pathology and x-ray results) and document patient care, but effective application of ICT also allows nurses to search for the best available research to inform their practice, and to support their clinical decisions with sound evidence (Levett-Jones et al. 2009). The use of ICT also supports the educational clinical needs of health professionals and clients who live in rural and remote areas.

Despite the obvious benefits of ICT in healthcare not all nurses or, indeed, nursing students have the confidence and competence needed to work with these technologies. Although most students quickly become familiar and confident with ICT, for some the requirement to use ICT, even in university settings, causes initial anxiety and stress, as the following quote shows:

> I just felt overwhelmed, panicked ... I thought, I can't do this ... I don't even know how to log on to the computer.
>
> (Levett-Jones et al. 2009)

Of particular significance is that some students do not recognise the relevance of ICT to clinical practice, and not all are aware that ICT skills can make a difference to the quality of patient care. The following comments illustrate this perspective:

> I can't see the point in all this ICT and online learning ... I wanted to do nursing ... not computer studies.
>
> ...
>
> Nurses want to work with people and learn from people ... I don't see how using ICT fits in at all.
>
> (Levett-Jones et al. 2009)

In clinical practice the use of ICT is sometimes regarded as the antithesis of therapeutic practice and in opposition to caring—the core concept of nursing. However, 'if nurses endeavour to overcome the barriers that technology presents to touch and meaningful human interactions, the patient's psychosocial needs will still be met in a person-centred way' (Timmins 2003).

Despite the concerns raised by some students and nurses, the increased use of ICT in education and in healthcare is inevitable. For more than 10 years the Australian Government has emphasised this point. In 2002 ICT was recognised as imperative for sustainable education and innovative nursing practice (Heath et al. 2009). A more recent study commissioned by the Australian Nursing Federation recommended the development of ICT competency standards and their incorporation into all nursing programs (Foster & Bryce 2009).

For the vast majority of nurses ICT is now regarded simply as 'tools of the trade' and a way to enhance the quality of patient care and reduce adverse events.

Embrace the opportunities provided at university and in clinical practice to become skilled and comfortable using a wide range of ICT applications. If you feel apprehensive most universities offer courses designed to improve your skills and confidence levels; fellow students, friends and family members are often able to provide the type of immediate support that is helpful.

While ICT competence will be of enormous benefit to you in your nursing career, ultimately it is your patients who will benefit most. Reflect on the following comments by new graduate nurses:

> I look up my patient pathology results every shift ... how else do I know what my patient's needs are? And for the older patients who might have come in with an acute delirium or have had surgery ... I have no idea what their previous cognitive level is. By reading the Aged Care Assessment Team reports online I at least have a basic understanding of where they were at before surgery.
>
> ...
>
> As a new grad ... I might be looking up something to do with wound management or I might be looking up normal saline versus hypertonic saline and more often than not I will be looking up something that the other nurses didn't know either and it is a way of sharing information around the ward.
>
> (Bembridge et al. 2011)

TELEPHONES AND THE INTERNET

The use of telephones and the internet as communication tools in modern society has progressed rapidly. As telephones and the internet are essential for workplace communication, there are some guidelines that you should be aware of and clinical facilities have policies that govern their use. Ward or unit telephones and computers are the property of the healthcare institution and financial costs are associated with their use. Unless it is essential for you to make a personal phone call or to send an urgent email, remember that the telephones and computers are for business use only. Using a telephone for personal calls may prevent other healthcare staff from using it to give or receive information relevant to patient care. Similarly, spending time on the ward computer prevents others from using it for more important patient-care purposes.

When you start on each new ward, ask what the policies are regarding telephone and internet access. In some facilities students are not to answer telephones or to give out patient information, and in many situations internet access is restricted to staff only.

Telephone guidelines

When you use the telephone you'll be expected to use appropriate telephone etiquette. This includes:

- answering the telephone promptly
- beginning the conversation with your name, designation and location
- discontinuing any conversation or activity before answering the telephone (e.g. eating or typing) and avoiding walking and talking while on the phone
- speaking clearly and distinctly, using a pleasant and professional tone of voice
- informing the caller when you are putting them on 'hold' and pressing the 'hold' button so they do not overhear other conversations that may be held close to the locality of the phone
- telling callers what your actions will be before you undertake them (e.g. 'I am going to transfer you to another number')
- always being courteous, friendly and ready to assist the caller
- passing on messages promptly—it is best to write the messages down rather than relying on your memory
- following facility requirements for telephone medication orders.

A mobile phone is now far more than just a telephone and is often referred to as a multimedia device with wireless connectivity. In the clinical learning environment a mobile phone has the potential to cause interference with technological equipment, and most health institutions request you to turn your mobile phone off as you enter. Your use of mobile phones during placement needs to be carefully considered. Making and receiving calls or text messaging should be done only in your breaks, if urgent. You will be expected to leave your mobile phone in your bag or locker and not carry it with you. You should also take care when using your phone as a multimedia device. Consider the following scenario.

STUDENT STORY
'They were only to help me remember'
Nikos' story

Nikos had been allocated to the special care nursery for his clinical placement. He was very excited and enthusiastic about this placement because it was an area he had selected for his graduate year. During the course of his placement, Nikos came across a baby who had a severe birth deformity. To help him to remember the condition, he took a series of photos using his mobile phone so he could add them to his professional portfolio.

At his debrief session, Nikos shared the photos with the other students and his clinical educator. Nikos had not sought written consent to take photos of the baby, and by using his mobile phone in this way he had unknowingly contravened the educational and healthcare institutions' policies as well as a number of laws related to privacy and confidentiality.

- Develop a courteous and effective telephone etiquette. Speak clearly and not too fast.
- Be mindful of the type of information you can divulge, and to whom, over the telephone in your role as a student.
- Always find out details about the person you are speaking to at the beginning of the call.
- Know the protocols for taking patient-care orders, test results and medication orders over the phone and adhere to these conventions strictly (see Box 5.4).
- Always put the principles of confidentiality and privacy into practice when answering telephones or using mobile devices during placement.
- Send and check text messages only in your breaks.
- Leave your placement location details (ward phone number) with your significant other in case of an emergency.
- Keep your contact details up to date in your university student records—telephone and email are sometimes used by lecturers to contact you.

Box 5.4	Telephone order guidelines

- When phoning a doctor, be organised. Have the information about the patient ready so you can answer any questions.
- Make sure you are aware of the patient's clinical condition, recent vital signs and other assessments before you make the call.
- Structure the phone call using the acronym ISBAR.
- When receiving phone orders use clarifying questions to avoid misunderstandings.
- Clearly determine the name, room number and diagnosis of the patient who you are discussing.
- Repeat any prescribed orders back to the doctor.
- Follow agency policies; most require telephone (and verbal) orders to be heard and signed by two nurses.
- Document the telephone order, including the date and time, the name of nurse(s) and doctor and the complete order.
- Have the doctor co-sign the order within the timeframe required by the institution (usually 24 hours).

Source: Crisp & Taylor 2012

USE OF SOCIAL MEDIA

Social media is changing the nature and speed of healthcare interactions between patients, health professionals and health organisations. Research indicates that 24% of patients interact with their health providers using social media, post about their healthcare experiences, provide reviews of their medications, and share health-related videos or images (PWC Health Industries 2014). Across the healthcare industry, from large hospital networks to patient support groups, social media tools like blogs, wikis, podcasts, instant messaging, video chat and social networks are reengineering the way health professionals and patients interact. Given the rapid changes in the communication landscape brought about by social media, it is important for nursing students to have a solid understanding of these technologies and their impact on health communication.

The increasing use of social media as a means of communication presents many legal and ethical issues in nursing education and clinical practice. What might be considered harmless chat or gossip has, when posted using social media, too often led to disciplinary processes, legal proceedings, exclusion from university and termination of employment. Derogatory comments about fellow students, patients, staff or healthcare institutions when discussed in social media sites such as Facebook or Twitter are considered to be unprofessional and a breach of university codes of conduct. The NMBA (2014) recently issued a social media policy to help nurses understand their obligations when using social media. The New Zealand Nursing Council (2012) also provides guidelines for social media. Additionally, you should keep in mind that social networking websites are being used by some employers and recruiters to screen potential employees. In the United States, for example, it is claimed that 45% of employers conduct these types of screening processes.

SOMETHING TO THINK ABOUT

How often do nurses breach professional guidelines and privacy laws in using social media?

- 27% of nurses admit to using social media to share stories about working life
- 41% of nurses say colleagues from their ward have used social media inappropriately
- 32% of these posts contained information about patients
- 12% of the posts contained photographs of patients

Source: Anonymous 2011

Coaching tips

Laurie Bickhoff is a newly graduated registered nurse and member of the Australian College of Nursing's Emerging Nurse Leader program. She writes extensively about nurses' use of social media. Laurie's coaching tips for using social media include:

- Everything you post should be considered public. If you wouldn't shout it at the supermarket you shouldn't post it online.
- Know that anything you post on social media reflects directly on the professionalism of all nurses. It is not just your reputation that is at risk but that of our colleagues, the ward and the healthcare organisation as well.

Coaching tips (cont'd)

- Think before posting—would you be comfortable if your patient, lecturers, boss, family, the Australian Health Practitioner Regulation Agency (AHPRA) or the police saw what you had posted?

- A breach of social media etiquette constitutes immoral and unethical behaviour; it is a breach of patient privacy laws and a breach of professional standards.

- Maintain confidentiality at all times—ensure patients and other people cannot be identified in your posts without their consent.

- Avoid defamation (i.e. unfounded or misinformed reports about someone).

- Maintain privacy—your own as well as your patients and colleagues. Use password protection and in-built privacy and safety features.

- Know the social media policy at your university and workplace.

- Consider how you would feel if the post was about your or someone you care about.

- Don't post photographs of yourself engaging in activities that you know would be deemed inappropriate by the nursing profession or by your university.

- Don't make comments on your website that bring your university or clinical placement venues into disrepute.

- Ensure any photos taken in a workplace and posted on social media sites meet legal and ethical standards (i.e. confidentiality, privacy, informed consent).

Source: Bickhoff 2013

SOMETHING TO THINK ABOUT

The social media post below was posted by a nursing student. Consider how you would feel if the post was about someone you care about.

F@*K! If they give me that smelly old guy with wrinkly genitals who won't speak English to wash again … I swear I'll just walk out and not come back!

SELF-DISCLOSURE

Self-disclosure is an act of revelation. What should you reveal about yourself in the course of your placement and to whom? Should you share your medical history or personal problems with your clients?

While there might be rare occasions when self-disclosure may be appropriate, it should always be well thought-out and not done to satisfy your own needs (e.g. to gain sympathy or attention). Before you engage in self-disclosure, reflect on your own agenda and motivation. Is your self-disclosure a genuine act to help others or a way to satisfy your own needs?

Some clinical placements provide the opportunity for you to attend group meetings. During these meetings clients often disclose personal information about themselves, and at times you may be tempted to share your own experiences about a similar problem. Be cautious! The invitation by the group leader to be a part of the group is in your capacity as a nursing student. It is not for you to discuss your personal circumstances, health conditions or life history. The intention is for you to learn from the group discussions and to focus on the therapeutic interactions that occur. In group meetings attention should not be drawn away from the clients.

The same principles apply if you have the opportunity to be involved in a case conference. Objective, informed discussion that focuses on the clients is the purpose of the meetings. Don't be tempted to disclose personal information about yourself, even if it seems relevant. Be aware of where boundary violations may occur (NMBA 2008; New Zealand Nurses Organisation 2010).

Coaching tips

- Before you join a group counselling session, seek guidelines from the group leader about your role in group meetings.
- Show respect and listen attentively to all members of the group.
- Arrive on time for the group session and wait until the end to leave.
- Avoid talking to fellow students during a group therapy session. The focus is on the patients. Short conversations with a colleague are viewed as disrespectful and can often make patients or other group members angry.
- Do not disclose any personal information. This includes your medical, psychological or personal history.
- Save questions until after the meeting—it is not a question and answer session.
- Always thank the group members for allowing you to participate in their session.
- Ensure you maintain confidentiality after the session and do not discuss anything revealed by group members.

RECEIVING AND PROVIDING EFFECTIVE FEEDBACK

Effective feedback is an important component of student learning (Archer 2010) both during and following clinical placements (Cees 2012). Feedback, effectively delivered and thoughtfully received, has the potential to facilitate improvement and personal and professional growth (Rudland et al. 2013). Effective feedback processes provide information about past performance and strategies for future learning. The degree to which feedback facilitates change, learning and future performance depends on many factors, including the perception and acceptance of the feedback by the recipient, the way feedback is conveyed and the personal characteristics of those involved. Feedback should not be viewed as a bureaucratic process or a tool for control. It is not about being punitive but an opportunity to develop insights and self-awareness. Quality feedback enhances self-esteem and motivates learning. Reflect carefully and thoughtfully on the feedback you receive, and use it to improve your future performance (see the sections on reflective practice and on seeking feedback in Chapter 4).

Mechanisms for providing feedback may be formal, informal, formative or summative (Hung et al. 2012). Formal feedback mechanisms may include hard-copy or online appraisal documents that incorporate a rating scale, or forms that request open-ended comments. Informal feedback may be conversations that occur between you and your mentor regularly about your placement experience and clinical performance. Formative feedback does not accrue marks or a grade but consists of activities designed to determine a student's level of skill or knowledge and advice and strategies for improvement. Summative feedback generally accrues a mark or a grade and provides a final result for a student's academic or clinical performance. Regardless of the feedback provided it should be timely and specific. Another term that is gaining popularity is 'feeding forward'; this approach places greater emphasis on providing direction and advice that will improve future performance.

Feedback on student performance

You should expect to receive regular feedback from the nurses you work with and from your educator. This may be in the form of a formal evaluation of your clinical performance or as opportunistic feedback that provides you with immediate information about your performance of a specific task or situation.

Feedback needs to be given in an environment conducive to listening and comprehending (quiet and away from the distraction of other people) and at a time when you can pay attention to what is being said. Your willingness to accept and to respond to the feedback is an important factor in the feedback process. Listen attentively, reflect on what is said and be willing to discuss the issues presented. Mature negotiation skills will allow you to seek and qualify information. Ask for examples to illustrate a particular criterion. Be proactive and ask for strategies that will help you develop further. Your feedback session is not the time to bring up complaints about individuals. Issues of this kind should be dealt with at the time they occur. Most institutions have a mechanism for handling complaints or for commending someone.

Providing feedback on your placement experience

While you may receive feedback about your clinical performance, you may also be requested to provide constructive feedback about your clinical experiences, your mentor or your clinical educator. Your feedback needs to be carefully considered, given freely and with the intent to inform and to be honest. For feedback to be most effective, it should be provided immediately following your placement so you most accurately capture your thoughts, feelings and ideas. Informal and spontaneous feedback is also a valuable mechanism to affirm and value others.

- Be receptive to feedback about your performance. Actively strive to grow and develop from constructively offered feedback.

- Be willing to provide constructive, timely and specific feedback and to support quality mechanisms and processes. Remember that your feedback has the power to change practices and is therefore a critical component of your professional life.

- Remember to 'sandwich' your feedback: positive comments— then negative—finishing with positive.

- Think carefully about the type and tone of the feedback you provide to others and about your placement.

References

Anonymous. *Nurses breaching online rules. Nursing Times.net*. Online. Available: <http://search.proquest.com.ezproxy.uow.edu.au/docview/879432543/abstract?accountid=15112>; 2011 Accessed 02.03.14.

Archer JC. State of the science in health professional education: effective feedback. *Med Educ*. 2010;44(1): 101-108.

Australian Bureau of Statistics. *Doctors and nurses*. Online. Available: <http://www.abd.gov.au?AUSSTATS/abs@.nsf/Lookup/4102.0Main+Feature>; 2013 Accessed 15.03.14.

Australian Commission on Safety and Quality in Health Care. *Electronic medication management systems: a guide to safer implementation*. Online. Available: <http://www.safetyandquality.gov.au/our-work/medication-safety/electronic-medication-management-systems>; 2013 Accessed 01.03.14.

Australian Medical Association. *AMA clinical handover guide: safe handover, safe patients*. Online. Available: <https://ama.com.au/ama-clinical-handover-guide-safe-handover-safe-patients>; 2007 Accessed 01.03.14.

Bembridge E, Levett-Jones T, Jeong S. The transferability of information and communication technology skills from university to the workplace: a qualitative descriptive study. *Nurse Educ Today*. 2011;31(3):245-252.

Bickhoff L. Think before you tweet. *Nurs Rev*. 2013;9(10):29-32.

Buresh B, Gordon S. *From silence to voice. What nurses know and must communicate to the public*. New York: ILR Press; 2013.

Cees PM. The process of feedback in workplace-based assessment: organisation, delivery, continuity. *Med Educ*. 2012;46(6):604-612.

Crisp J, Taylor C, eds. *Potter and Perry's fundamentals of nursing*. 4th ed. Sydney: Mosby Elsevier; 2012.

Day J, Levett-Jones T, Kenny R. Communication. In: Berman A, Synder S, Levett-Jones T, et al., eds. *Kozier and Erb's fundamentals of nursing*. 2nd ed. Sydney: Pearson; 2015.

Dickson C. *The nature of learning to nurse through clinical practice experience for international culturally and linguistically different students in Sydney, Australia: an interpretive description*. Doctor of Nursing thesis. Sydney: University of Technology; 2013.

Foster J, Bryce J. Australian nursing informatics competency project. In: *Proceedings of the 10th International Congress on Nursing Informatics: Connecting Health and Humans, 28 June—1 July 2009*. Helsinki; 2009. Online. Available: <http://eprints.qut.edu.au/31927/1/c31927a.pdf>; Accessed 28.05.14.

Gardner A, Goodsell J, Duggen T, et al. 'Don't call me sweetie!' Patients differ from nurses in their perceptions of caring. *Collegian*. 2001;8(3):32-38.

Garling P. *Final report to the Special Commission of Inquiry. Acute care services in NSW Public Hospitals. Overview*. Online. Available: <www.lawlink.nsw.gov.au/acsinquiry>; 2008 Accessed 29.02.14.

Grice T. *Everyday English for nursing*. Edinburgh: Elsevier; 2003.

Hally M. *A guide for international nursing students in Australia and New Zealand*. Sydney: Churchill Livingstone Elsevier; 2009.

Harms L. *Working with people*. South Melbourne: Oxford University Press; 2007.

Heath P, Duncan J, Lowe E, et al. *National review of nursing education: our duty of care*. Online. Available: <http://www.dest.gov.au/archive/highered/nursing/pubs/duty_of_care/default.html>; 2009 Accessed 28.01.14.

Hung D, Lee S, Lim K. Authenticity in learning for the twenty-first century: bridging the formal and the informal. *Educ Technol Res Dev* [serial online]. 2012;60(6):1071-1091.

Iedema R. Handover. In: Levett-Jones T, ed. *Critical conversations for patient safety: an essential guide for health professionals.* Sydney: Pearson; 2014.

Inquest into the death of Vanessa Anderson. Sydney, Australia: Coroner's Court, Westmead; 2004.

Joint Commission. Sentinel events statistics. In: Leonard M, Graham S, Bonacum D, eds. The human factor: the critical importance of effective teamwork and communication in providing safe care. *Qual Saf Health Care.* 2004;13:i85-i90.

Jones SS, Rudin RS, Perry T, et al. Health information technology. An updated systematic review with a focus on meaningful use. *Ann Intern Med.* 2014;160(1):48-54.

Lapkin S, Levett-Jones T, Gilligan C. *The development and testing of the Theory of Planned Behaviour Medication Safety Questionnaire. Nurse Educ Today.* in press.

Levett-Jones T. *Critical conversations for patient safety: an essential guide for health professionals.* Sydney: Pearson; 2014.

Levett-Jones T, Kenny R, Van der Riet P, et al. Exploring the information and communication technology competence and confidence of nursing students and their perception of its relevance to clinical practice. *Nurse Educ Today.* 2009;29(6):612-616.

Levett-Jones T, Oates K, MacDonald-Wicks L. The relationship between communication and patient safety. In: Levett-Jones T, ed. *Critical conversations for patient safety: an essential guide for health professionals.* Sydney: Pearson; 2014.

Morse J, Proctor A. Maintaining patient endurance: the comfort work of trauma nurses. *Clin Nurs Res.* 1998; 7(3):250-274.

National Health and Hospitals Reform Commission. *A healthier future for all Australians—Final Report of the National Health and Hospitals Reform Commission—June 2009. 2009.* Online. Available: <http://www.health .gov.au/internet/nhhrc/publishing.nsf/Content/1AFDEAF1FB76A1D8CA257600000B5BE2/$File/EXEC _SUMMARY.pdf>; 2009 Accessed 29.01.14.

New Zealand Nurses Organisation. *Standards of professional nursing practice.* Online. Available: <www.nzno.org .nz/resources/nzno_publications>; 2010 Accessed 16.01.14.

New Zealand Nursing Council. *Guidelines: social media and electronic communication.* Online. Available: <www .nzno.org.nz/resources/nzno_publications>; 2012 Accessed 16.01.14.

Nursing and Midwifery Board of Australia (NMBA). *National competency standards for the registered nurse.* Online. Available: <www.nursingmidwiferyboard.gov.au>; 2006 Accessed 16.01.14.

Nursing and Midwifery Board of Australia (NMBA). *Code of professional conduct for nurses in Australia.* Online. Available: <www.nursingmidwiferyboard.gov.au>; 2008 Accessed 01.03.14.

Nursing and Midwifery Board of Australia (NMBA). *Social media policy.* Online. Available: <www .nursingmidwiferyboard.gov.au>; 2014 Accessed 01.03.14.

OECD. *International migration of health workers: improving international cooperation to address the global health worker crisis.* Online. Available: <http://www.oecd.org/dataoecd/8/1/44783473.pdf>;2010 Accessed 15.03.14.

PWC Health Industries. *Social media 'likes' healthcare: from marketing to social business.* Online. Available: <http://www.pwc.com/us/en/health-industries/publications/health-care-social-media.jhtml>; 2014 Accessed 15.03.14.

Rossiter R, Scott R, Walton C. Key attributes of therapeutic communication. In: Levett-Jones T, ed. *Critical conversations for patient safety: an essential guide for health professionals.* Sydney: Pearson; 2014.

Rudland J, Wilkinson T, Wearn A, et al. A student-centred feedback model for educators. *Clin Teach.* 2013;10(2):99-102.

Rungby J, Brock B. What can we do to improve adherence in patients with diabetes? In: Barnett AH, ed. *Clinical challenges in diabetes.* Oxford: Atlas Medical Publishing; 2010.

Sonneman V. *Existence and therapy: an introduction to phenomenological psychology and existential analysis.* New York: Grune & Stratton; 1959.

Swift A. *Honesty and ethics rating of clergy slides to new low. Nurses are again top list; lobbyists are worst. Gallup Politics 16 Dec 2013.* Online. Available: <http://www.gallup.com/poll/166298/honesty-ethics-rating-clergy -slides-new-low.aspx>; 2013 Accessed 01.03.14.

Timmins J. Nurses resisting information technology. *Nurs Inq.* 2003;10(4):257-269.

Trede F, Ellis E, Jones S. Communication and duty of care. In: Higgs J, Ajjawi R, McAllister L, et al., eds. *Communicating in the health sciences.* 3rd ed. South Melbourne: Oxford University Press; 2012.

Tsai J, Bond G. A comparison of electronic records to paper records in mental health centers. *Int J Qual Health Care.* 2008;20(2):136.

Wong M, Yee K, Turner P. *A structured evidence-based literature review regarding effectiveness of improvement interventions in clinical handover. Australia: eHealth Services Research Group, University of Tasmania/ACSQHC; 2008.* Online. Available: <www.achs.health.nsw.gov.au/clHoverLitReview.pdf>; 2008 Accessed 30.01.14.

GLOSSARY

Accountability
Relates to the forms of responsibility and duty, and to the notion of 'being in charge of' in nursing practice.

Acculturation
The individual's adaptation to the customs, values, beliefs and behaviours of a new culture.

Acuity
The degree of complexity of a patient's state of illness and the level of care required.

Advocacy
A critical function of the nursing role that incorporates the ethical principle of beneficence, defending the rights of others or acting on their behalf.

Ageism
Prejudice against older adults that perpetuates negative stereotyping of ageing as a period of decline.

Androgogy
The art and science of helping adults learn; a term coined by Malcolm Knowles to describe his theory of adult learning (1984).

Assess
To gather, summarise and interpret relevant data about a learner or patient to make a decision or plan.

Best practice
The use of high-quality clinical evidence to inform and underpin patient-care decisions and nursing actions.

Clinical educator
The registered nurse assigned to facilitate student learning. A clinical educator is usually allocated to a group of students, and may or may not be employed by the educational institution; also called facilitator, clinical teacher and nurse teacher.

Clinical governance
A system of management that encourages openness about strengths and weaknesses, and that incorporates the need to be proactive through best practice to promote excellence in healthcare.

Clinical learning environment
The placement location in a healthcare facility where nursing students are allocated in order to achieve objectives, care for clients/patients and undertake assigned learning activities.

Clinicians and other health professionals
The nurses who work with patients/clients in the clinical learning environment.

Code of Ethics for Nurses in Australia
A framework that outlines the nursing profession's intention to accept the rights of individuals and to uphold these rights in practice. The code provides guidelines for ethical practice and identifies the fundamental moral commitments of the nursing profession.

Code of Professional Conduct for Nurses in Australia
A set of national standards of nursing conduct for nurses in Australia that identifies the minimum requirements for conduct in the profession.

Competence
The combination of knowledge, skills, behaviours, attitudes, values and abilities that underpins effective and/or superior performance in a professional or occupational area.

Compliance
Submission or yielding to regimens or practices prescribed or established by others.

Confidentiality
A binding social contract or covenant; a professional obligation to respect privileged information between a health provider and client/patient.

Cultural competence
The ability to demonstrate knowledge and understanding of another person's culture, and accept and respect cultural differences by adapting interventions to be congruent with that specific culture when delivering care.

Culture
A complex concept that is an integral part of each person's life. It includes knowledge, beliefs, values, morals, customs, traditions and habits acquired by the members of a society.

Disability
Inability to perform some key functions of living.

Duty
Responsibility; professional expectation.

Educational institution
An institution that provides an accredited nursing program. The institution may be a university, school of nursing or college.

Educator
The teaching role a nurse assumes in supporting, encouraging and assisting a learner.

Enrolled nurse
A person licensed to provide nursing care under the supervision of a registered nurse.

Ethical dilemma
A problem in which there is a moral or ethical choice to be made between options that seem equally unfavourable.

Ethics
Guiding principles of human behaviour; morals.

Ethnicity
A dynamic and complex concept referring to how members of a group perceive themselves and how, in turn, they are perceived by others in relation to the population subgroup's common heritage of customs, characteristics, language and history.

Ethnocentrism
The belief that one's own culture is superior and all other cultures are less sophisticated.

Feedback
Valid and reliable judgements about students' performance for the purposes of recognising strengths and areas for improvement. Feedback provides students with information about what they are expected to do and how they are progressing.

Ideally, it is provided about all activities or situations in which the student has been involved.

Healthcare facility
An institution in which the delivery of healthcare is the primary focus. Examples include hospitals, outpatient clinics, medical centres and extended care facilities. These may be publicly or privately operated.

Healthcare team
An interdisciplinary group of healthcare professionals and non-professionals who provide services to patients and their families in an attempt to maximise the optimal health and wellbeing of the person to whom their activities are directed.

Horizontal violence
Covert or overt dissatisfaction directed by nurses towards one another and towards those less powerful than themselves. Usually it is the nurses in the least organisationally powerful positions that manifest bullying among themselves and towards those with even less power. Sometimes referred to as workplace bullying.

International nursing student
A student undertaking an approved nursing course or program who is not an Australian citizen and is not permanently residing in Australia.

Interprofessional healthcare team
The different disciplinary groups of people responsible for working as a team to provide high-quality healthcare to patients.

Learning objectives
Intended outcomes of the educational process that are action-oriented rather than content-oriented, and learner-centred rather than teacher-centred.

Mentor
A nurse who supports a nursing student during a placement experience. The nurse takes responsibility for supervising, directly or indirectly, the student's practice. Sometimes referred to as a preceptor, buddy or professional partner or allocated registered nurse.

Negligence
Doing or not doing an act, pursuant to a duty, that a reasonable person in the same circumstances would or would not do, and that results in injury to another person.

Nursing and Midwifery Board of Australia (NMBA) Competency Standards for the Registered Nurse (2006)
A national benchmark for registered nurses that reinforces responsibility and accountability in delivering quality nursing care through safe and effective work practice. The competencies are organised into four domains: professional practice; critical thinking and analysis; provision and coordination of care; and collaborative and therapeutic practice.

Person-centred care
A way of practising that focuses on an individual's personal beliefs, values, wants, needs and desires. An approach in which person's freedom to make their own decisions is recognised as a fundamental and valuable human right.

Privacy
A right for all individuals that protects their personal information and the dissemination of such information.

Reflection
A process by which nurses assess their clinical experience and their understanding of what they are doing and why they are doing it, and consider the impact it has on themselves and others. Reflection promotes learning from practice through

exploration, questioning and growing through, and as a consequence of, clinical experiences.

Registered nurse
A person who is licensed to practise nursing in Australia.

Scope of practice
A framework of nursing activities that particular nurses are educated, competent and authorised to perform within a specific context.

Sexual harassment
Conduct of a sexual nature that is unwanted and unwelcome by the receiver. Conduct is considered unwelcome when it is neither invited nor solicited and the behaviour is deemed offensive and undesirable.

Student
A student of nursing may be an undergraduate nursing student or a trainee enrolled nurse.

Undergraduate nursing program
An initial program of study that leads to the award of a bachelor's degree and is provided at institutions of higher education (usually universities but may be institutes or approved colleges).

INDEX

Page numbers followed by 'f' indicate figures, 't' indicate tables, and 'b' indicate boxes.